# A STUDY OF

# SHIATSU

## CASS & JANIE JACKSON

Acknowledgments
Special thanks to:
Michelle Wattam, Shiatsu practitioners Dip. B.S.S. M.R.S.S.
and Vivienne Isaac for their professional services, advice and guidance.
The Glenmore Centre, Shepshed,
for the use of their excellent facilities.
The Helix Centre, Loughborough.
Charles Walker Photographic: p.14-15, p.46, p.47


Published in 2002 by Caxton Editions
20 Bloomsbury Street
London WC1B 3JH
a member of the Caxton Publishing Group


© 2002 Caxton Publishing Group


Designed and produced for Caxton Editions
by Open Door Limited
Rutland, United Kingdom


Editing: Mary Morton
Setting: Jane Booth
Digital Imagery © copyright 2002 PhotoDisc Inc.

Title: A Study of Shiatsu
ISBN: 1 84067 297 8

IMPORTANT NOTICE:
This book is not intended to be a substitute for medical
advice or treatment. Any person with a condition requiring
medical attention should consult a qualified medical
practitioner or therapist.

# A STUDY OF

# SHIATSU

## CASS & JANIE JACKSON

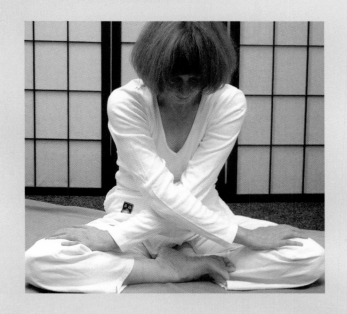

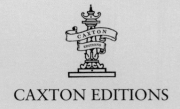

CAXTON EDITIONS

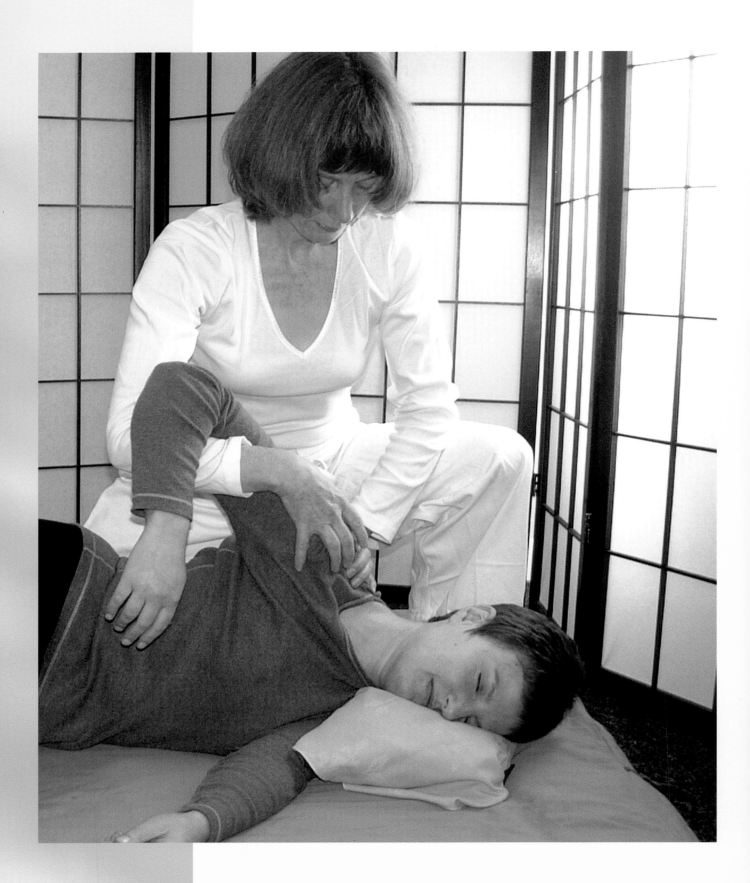

# CONTENTS

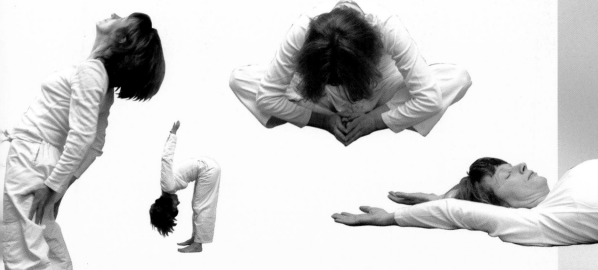

# INTRODUCTION

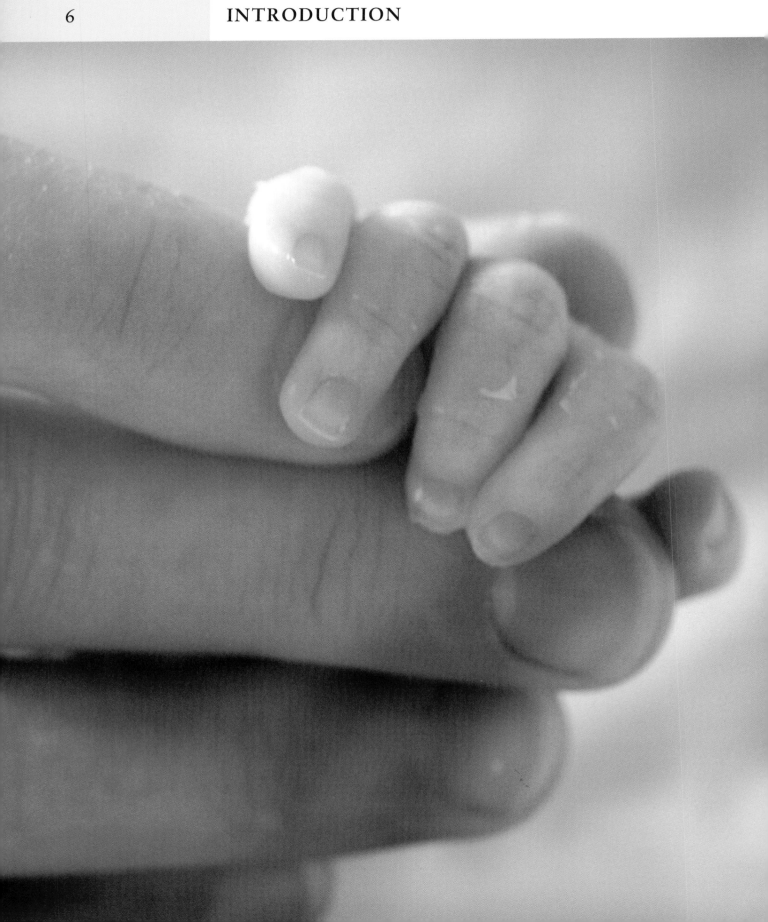

This book explains what Shiatsu is and how it works. It touches on the history and development of the therapy and explains its position in the world today.

Shiatsu's main function is to ensure the maintenance of a healthy body, thereby preventing illness, but it can also be used to treat a number of common maladies. Like most other Oriental therapies, too, it offers emotional, spiritual and mental benefits.

The actual techniques of Shiatsu are simple to apply, but newcomers to the therapy may find some difficulty in understanding the various terms used. Don't allow this to deter you. One section of this book is entitled THE LANGUAGE OF SHIATSU and it explains most of the unfamiliar words you will come across. This section will act as a valuable reference tool during your studies. You are advised to read it carefully before attempting any Shiatsu treatment.

At the same time, do understand that Shiatsu is meant to be relaxing and joyful. It is based on the power of touch – which we are aware of from the day we are born. In the past, the British "stiff upper lip" precluded physical contact among adults, particularly males. Fortunately, this attitude has changed. Nowadays, even tough guys like footballers hug

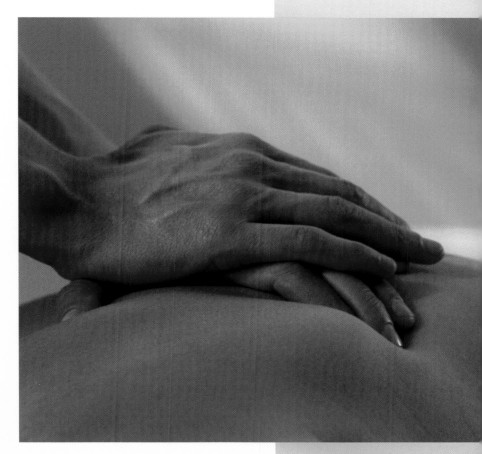

each other on the field and such behaviour is no longer unacceptable.

Touch is important to our emotional health. In Shiatsu it is applied in such a way that it affects every aspect of our well-being – body, mind and spirit. Learning to use this ancient therapy will open the door to many new experiences and – if you wish – it will change your life.

*Above: touch is important to our emotional health. In Shiatsu it is applied in such a way that it affects every aspect of our well-being – body, mind and spirit.*

*Far left: Shiatsu is based on the power of touch – which we are aware of from the day we are born.*

# WHAT IS SHIATSU?

S HIATSU is a Japanese healing art and this book offers a simple introduction to it.

Literally translated Shiatsu means "finger pressure", and these two words define the basis of the procedure.

## THE JAPANESE STYLE

The Japanese style of Shiatsu – introduced into the West some 30 years ago – was a fairly dynamic affair, causing a lot of discomfort and sometimes quite severe pain. At one time, the popular concept of a Shiatsu treatment was that the practitioner walked up and down the client's back. Unfortunately, some people still have this image of what Shiatsu involves.

## TIMES HAVE CHANGED

In fact, Western practitioners have greatly modified the Japanese style and today – though it can still cause some brief discomfort – Shiatsu is a much more gentle affair. The pressure involved comes mainly from the fingers, but the thumbs and palms are also used and, occasionally, the knees, the forearms. the elbows and the feet.

Shiatsu therapy works in various ways.

*Below: literally translated Shiatsu means "finger pressure".*

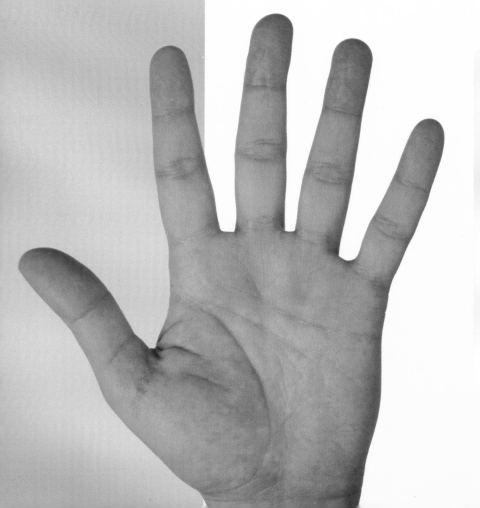

It clears toxins from the body.

It releases tensions from the muscles and joints.

It has a relaxing effect on the nervous system.

It stimulates the body's healing abilities.

It increases the circulation and promotes the flow of lymphatic fluid.

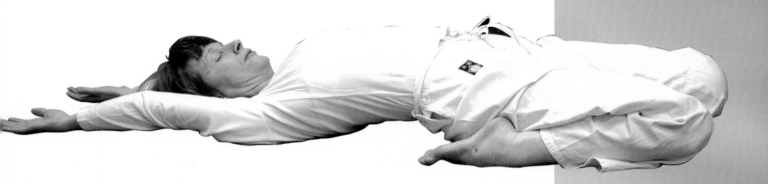

## NOT JUST A PHYSICAL THERAPY

Although treatment is based on the application of pressure, stretching, kneading the muscles and supporting the body, it is by no means a purely physical therapy. Shiatsu treatment is strictly "hands on". Consequently, it also demands close communication with other people and a strong desire to support and help them. At the end of a Shiatsu treatment session both client and practitioner should feel energised, relaxed and totally balanced.

## SELF DEVELOPMENT

A Shiatsu session does not always require the assistance of a qualified practitioner. Certain Shiatsu exercises and methods can be self-applied and, as with other holistic therapies such as Tai Chi and yoga, will have the effect of "grounding" body, mind and spirit.

Even if you never receive a Shiatsu treatment from a practitioner, you can benefit from a brief, daily self-help session. It is possible to learn the routine from books but, if at all possible, two or three introductory classes are advisable. Tell your tutor that you are planning to enjoy regular Shiatsu sessions at home and he/she will be happy to help you.

*Above: even if you never receive a Shiatsu treatment from a practitioner, you can benefit from a brief, daily self-help session.*

### ADVANTAGES

In Japan, Shiatsu is widely used as a family remedy and this is an aspect that is steadily gaining ground in the West. The therapy lends itself well to home use. No special equipment is needed, there is no need to remove clothing, and the movements are so simple that they can readily be mastered.

Additionally, of course, once you have learned the basic elements of Shiatsu, you will be able to use it to help other people. A number of everyday aches, pains and stresses can be alleviated quickly and easily. The power of touch can be incredibly relaxing, healing and strengthening, at both a physical and emotional level. What's more, both the giver and the recipient benefit from the exchange of energy. The result is invariably positive – it relieves stress, enhances a feeling of well-being, and strengthens relationships.

### BECOMING A PROFESSIONAL

Shiatsu can certainly be used in self-treatment, but the therapy can be extremely complex. It requires a great deal of dedication from those seeking to practise it professionally.

Becoming a Shiatsu practitioner involves a long period of dedicated study and practical work. The Shiatsu Society (see Appendix) sets extremely high standards for the practice of the therapy in the UK. It demands that all students wishing to be recognised by the Society should have spent a minimum of 500 hours of study with a registered teacher over a period of at least three years. Students may not apply to join the professional register until they have served their "apprenticeship" and, even then, they must be assessed before such recognition is granted.

*Below: in Japan, Shiatsu is widely used as a family remedy.*

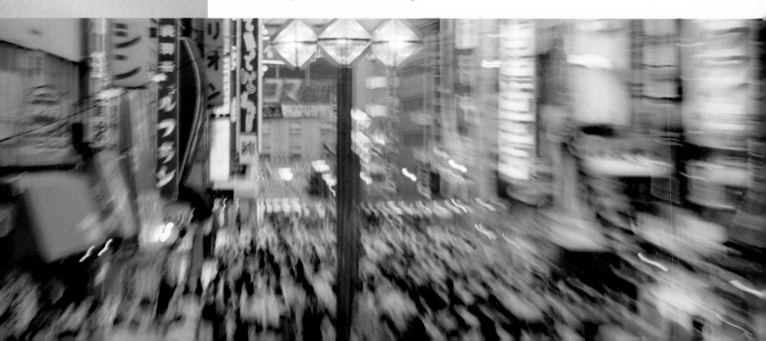

The name Shiatsu was not introduced until the early 20th century, but this healing art is firmly rooted in the Oriental traditions of medicine, probably originating in China some 500 years before the birth of Christ. Acupuncture, herbalism and several types of massage were essential techniques in Traditional Chinese Medicine (TCM) and gradually these methods spread from China to other parts of Asia.

By the 6th century AD, the Japanese had incorporated their own ideas into TCM and developed a therapy called anma. This was a type of massage that also involved the use of vibrational healing and acupressure.

For many years, anma was an integral part of medical training for Japanese doctors, used to establish their knowledge of the structure of the human body, energy channels and pressure points.

## BLIND MASSEURS

However, at some time during the 17th or 18th century, it was decreed that massage should be a profession for the blind, on the grounds that their lack of sight enhanced their sense of touch. This decision heralded a marked deterioration in the practice of anma.

Blind people, in general, were poorly educated, since no facilities existed to compensate for their disability. For this reason, many of the medical aspects of anma were lost or forgotten. In consequence, masseurs lacked the qualifications enjoyed by doctors and their status deteriorated. Anma came to be regarded almost as a recreational therapy; a pleasurable method for enhancing relaxation.

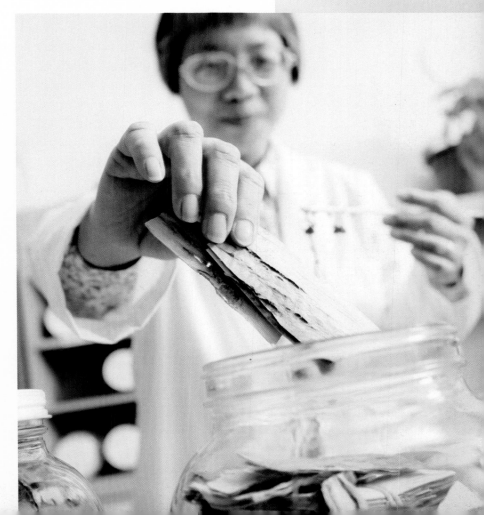

*Below: acupuncture, herbalism and several types of massage are essential techniques in Traditional Chinese Medicine.*

### REVIVAL

It was not until early in the 20th century that the situation began to change. Many practitioners of anma had continued to maintain the therapy's original high standards. They were further inspired, in 1919, by the publication of a book called *Shiatsu Ho* by Tamai Tempaku.

This man was an anma practitioner who had also studied Western theories of massage, anatomy and physiology. His book led directly to the establishment of several distinct forms of Shiatsu.

### NAMIKOSHI SHIATSU

One of these was introduced by Tokujiro Namikoshi. A devoted son, he originally used massage only to help his mother, who was arthritic. Eventually, he adopted the anma system, but continued to incorporate his own techniques.

In 1925 he opened a clinic at the Shiatsu Institute of Therapy in Hokkaido. Fifteen years later, he established the Japan Shiatsu Institute in Tokyo.

Namikoshi's approach to Shiatsu was designed to appeal to Westerners and he was particularly anxious to spread the news of the therapy to the USA. In consequence, he made no mention of traditional theories such as anma, meridians or energy. His techniques – which have been continued by his son, Toru Namikoshi – are basically physical with little reference to spiritual aspects.

### OFFICIAL RECOGNITION

Namikoshi must be credited with spreading information about Shiatsu to the West and with the official recognition of Shiatsu in Japan. In 1955 the therapy was

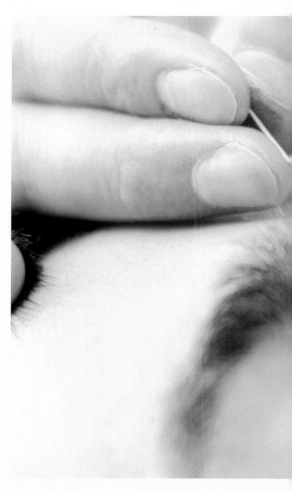

legally accepted as part of anma, and two years later Namikoshi's school was recognised by the Japanese government. But it was not until 1964 that Shiatsu was officially acknowledged in Japan as being a therapy in its own right.

## PROOF OF EXISTENCE

Another pioneer of Shiatsu in the form we know it today is Katsusuke Serizawa. Throughout his career, he concentrated his research on the tsubo – that is, the pressure points thought to exist at certain positions along the meridians. In Shiatsu, pressure is applied to stimulate these points; in acupuncture, needles are used.

Serizawa made a close study of the locations of the tsubo in traditional Oriental medicine. Then, using modern electrical methods, he tested the meridians and the tsubo. The results of his research enabled him to offer scientific proof of their existence. His work was rewarded with a Doctor of Medicine degree.

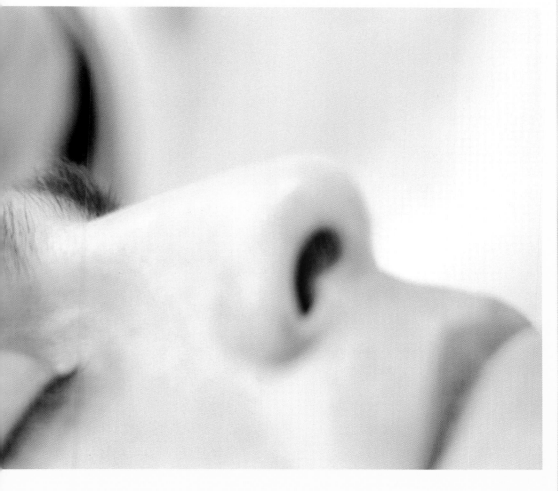

*Left: in Shiatsu, pressure is applied to stimulate the pressure points thought to exist at certain positions along the meridians – in acupuncture, needles are used.*

*Right: Ki lines, marked out on the human body. Masunaga returned Shiatsu to its traditional roots. He based his theories on TCM, and also employed a number of other techniques for manipulating the flow of energy throughout the body.*

### ACUPRESSURE SHIATSU

Serizawa called his treatment Tsubo Therapy. His method gives primary importance to the pressure points, using various traditional and contemporary methods of stimulation.

Although this style is slightly different from current Shiatsu practice, it is particularly popular in America, where it is known as Acupressure Shiatsu.

### SHIATSU IN THE WEST

The leading exponent of Shiatsu outside Japan was Shizuto Masunaga. His book – *Zen Shiatsu* – was published in 1977, since when his methods have become widely used in the West.

It was Masunaga who returned the therapy to its traditional roots. He based his theories on TCM, and also employed a number of other techniques for manipulating the flow of energy throughout the body. This style of treatment, known as Zen Shiatsu, is probably the most popular and widely used in the Western world. It is the style to which we refer most frequently in this book.

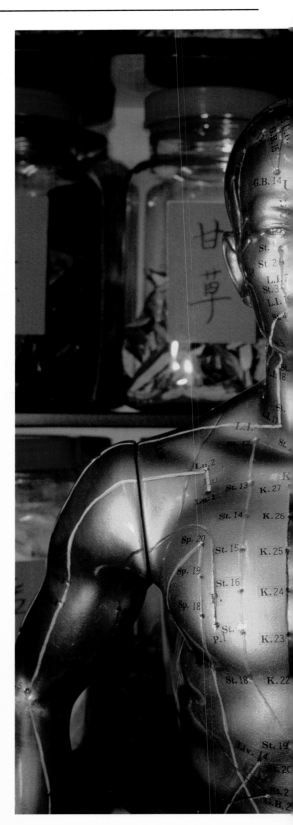

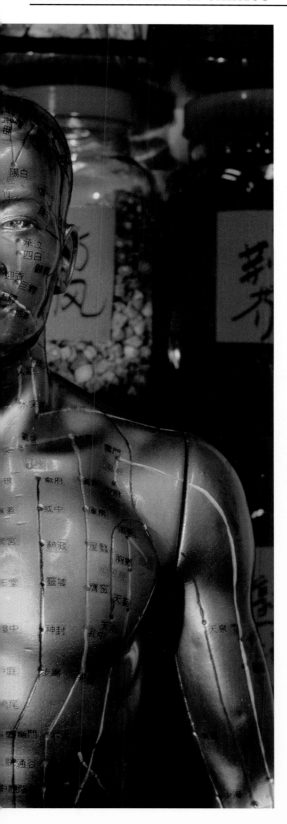

## OTHER TYPES OF SHIATSU

Since the publication of Masunaga's book and his introduction of Zen Shiatsu, a number of other developments have taken place. As with most complementary therapies, certain practitioners have advanced new theories and introduced their own distinctive styles. For example, Macrobiotic Shiatsu incorporates certain dietary rules – and Ohashiatsu blends the Zen method with those of Namikoshi. It is even possible to receive Shiatsu treatment in water, a method developed by a therapist in California.

There is not space here for even a cursory investigation into these Shiatsu styles, but more information is readily obtainable from the wide variety of books published on the subject. (See Appendix for suggestions.)

# THE LANGUAGE OF SHIATSU

This book is written as simply as possible in everyday language, but it still contains certain words that will be unfamiliar to the average reader. If you wish to learn more about Shiatsu – whether as a practitioner or merely from interest in the subject – you will come across still more of these unusual words. Listed below are some aspects of "Shiatsu talk" which may help you.

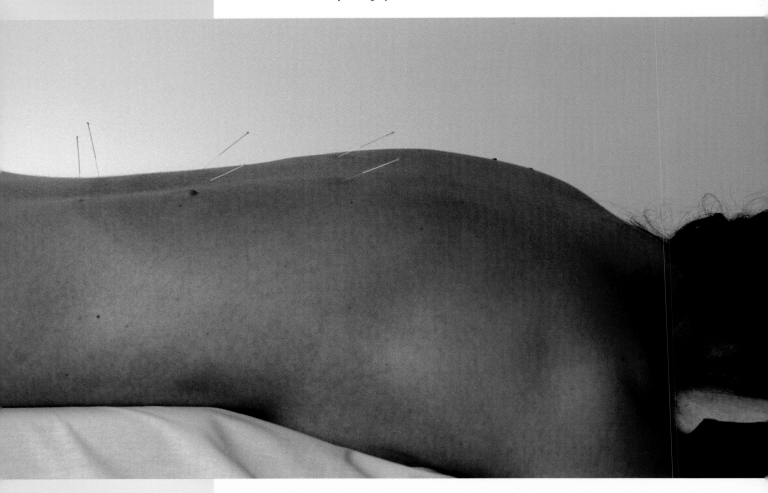

## ACUPRESSURE

As with Shiatsu, the aim of acupressure is to balance the flow of Ki. The same pressure points are used as in acupuncture, but no needles are involved. **Acupressure** is a part of Traditional Chinese Medicine (TCM).

## ACUPUNCTURE

The word **acupuncture** means, literally, "pricking with a needle". This treatment is also part of TCM and its aim is to restore the balance of Ki. During treatment, fine needles are inserted on the pressure points along the meridians.

## AHSHI POINTS

Any painful point on the body, not necessarily on a meridian, is called an **ahshi** point.

## AMPUKA

A specialised form of abdominal massage originating in Japan. It was used particularly for gynaecological problems and in childbirth.

## ANMA

This ancient form of massage incorporated vibrational healing, spot pressure and massage. Although it was originally considered part of medical training for Japanese doctors, it gradually came to be regarded only as a means of relaxation.

## CALMING

A Shiatsu technique used to calm and control agitated energy.

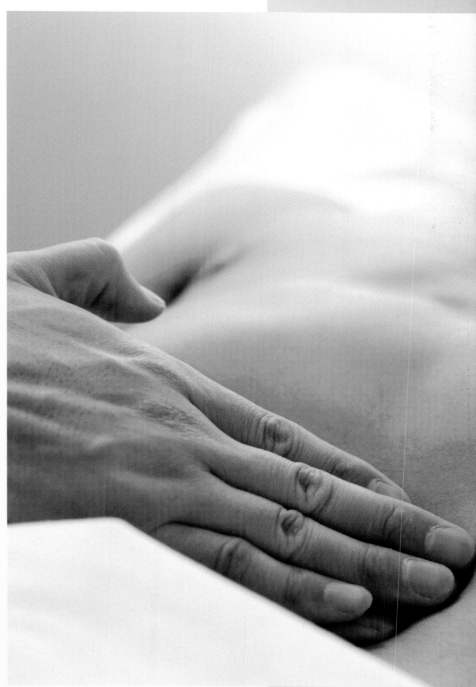

*Below: Ampuka – a form of abdominal massage.*

*Below: the Chakras.*

## CHAKRAS

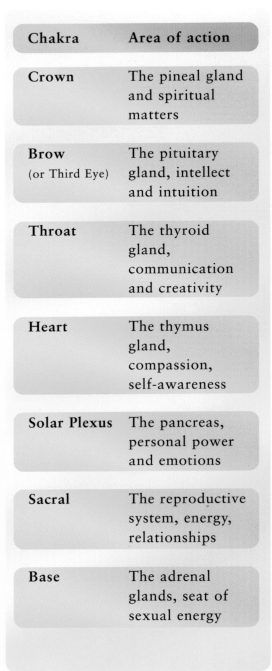

These seven main energy centres are located down the middle of the body. They are believed to be situated along the spiritual channel, which begins at the crown of the head and runs to the base of the trunk. Each chakra is associated with a specific area of action, thus:

| Chakra | Area of action |
| --- | --- |
| Crown | The pineal gland and spiritual matters |
| Brow (or Third Eye) | The pituitary gland, intellect and intuition |
| Throat | The thyroid gland, communication and creativity |
| Heart | The thymus gland, compassion, self-awareness |
| Solar Plexus | The pancreas, personal power and emotions |
| Sacral | The reproductive system, energy, relationships |
| Base | The adrenal glands, seat of sexual energy |

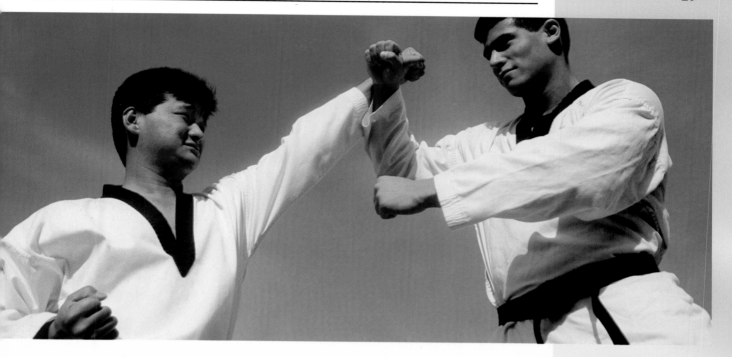

## CORRESPONDENCES

Each of the Five Elements is considered to possess certain characteristics similar to those of various parts of the body and emotions. These qualities are known as **correspondences**.

## CUN

The **cun** is the measurement concerned with the location of tsubo. It is a totally individual measurement, varying according to the size of the person, and is roughly the width of a thumb.

## DISPERSAL

Also known as "sedation", this Shiatsu technique is used to disperse blocked energy.

## DO-IN

An energising system of exercise, **Do-In** is traditionally used as a warm-up in martial arts. Many Shiatsu classes start with a Do-In session.

## DRAGON'S MOUTH

A Shiatsu technique using the webbing between the thumb and index finger, which is particularly suited to work on curved areas such as the arms. The digits are stretched wide (thus **dragon's mouth**), the main pressure being from the knuckle at the base of the index finger.

*Above: Do-In is traditionally used as a warm-up in martial arts. Many Shiatsu classes start with a Do-In session.*

*Right: Fu organs-produce energy from food and drink.*

*Far right: Jing governs growth, our ability to produce children and the ageing process.*

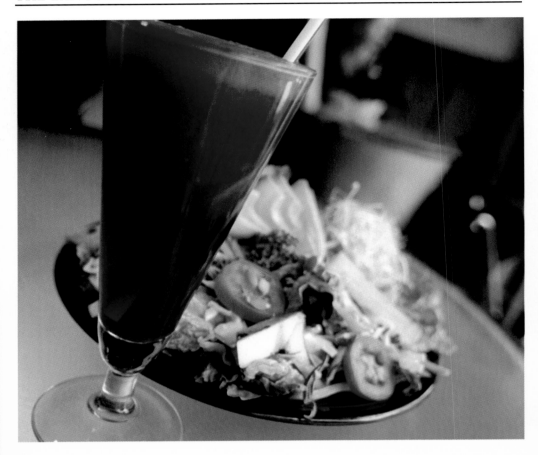

## FIVE ELEMENTS

This theory originated in TCM and provides an explanation of how energy (Ki) transforms from one state to another. The **Five Elements** are wood, fire, earth, metal and water.

## FU ORGANS

According to TCM, each organ of the body has two functions – one physical and one concerned with the use of energy. **Fu organs** (more commonly known as Yin) produce energy from food and drink and control excretion. See also **Yang organs**.

## FUTON

A **futon** is a mattress made from layers of cotton padding. It originated in Japan where it was used as a bed at night and, rolled up, as a seat during the day. Most Shiatsu practitioners provide a futon on which clients lie for treatment.

## HARA

**Hara** is the Japanese word for abdomen. It contains a vital energy centre known as the Tan Den, and is considered to be the major source of physical and spiritual strength.

## HEART GOVERNOR

Also known as the Heart Protector, the **Heart Governor** supports the functions of the heart, controls the circulation of blood and influences relationships.

## JING

This is the vital energy stored in the kidneys. It governs growth, our ability to produce children and the ageing process.

## KI

This is the Japanese word for "vital energy". In Shiatsu it is generally used to refer to the energy in the body. **Ki** is associated with a number of important functions, including the transformation of food into energy, the flow of fluids, and the protection of the body.

## KYO-JITSU

Though often used together, these two words have different meanings. **Kyo** means emptiness. **Jitsu** describes fullness or blockage in a meridian or tsubo. Thus, Kyo-Jitsu refers to the relative states of activity or lack of same within the channels.

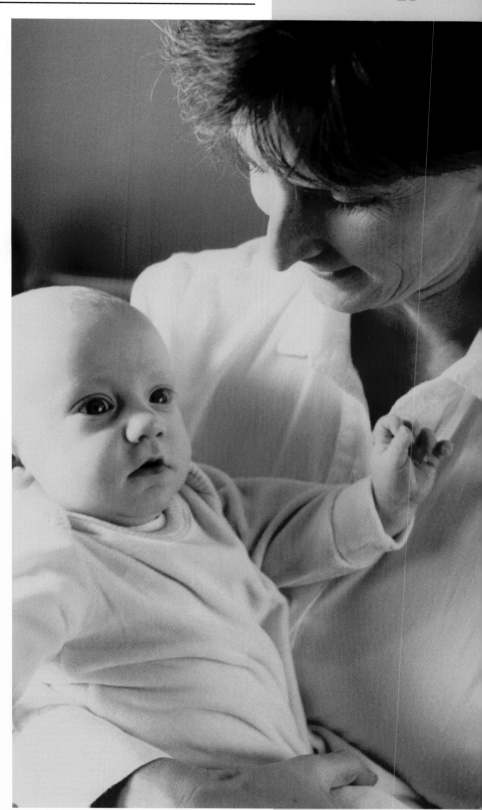

### MACROBIOTICS

A diet in which food is designated into Yin and Yang categories. Macrobiotic Shiatsu uses the traditional meridians but incorporates the dietary and lifestyle theories developed by Michio Kushi and George Ohsawa.

### MAKKO-HO

This special exercise system, devised by Shizuto Masunaga for Zen Shiatsu, enhances the flow of Ki throughout the body. It also maintains joint flexibility. Even if you are not practising Shiatsu, this is an excellent daily exercise routine for general fitness.

### MERIDIANS

These energy channels form a network allowing Ki to flow throughout the body. Each **meridian**, or channel, is associated with an internal organ and bears the same name.

### MOXIBUSTION

A technique used to promote healing where heat is required. Moxibustion involves the burning of mugwort on or above a specific point.

### SEDATION

See **Dispersal** above.

*Below: Moxibustion is the burning of mugwort on or above a specific point.*

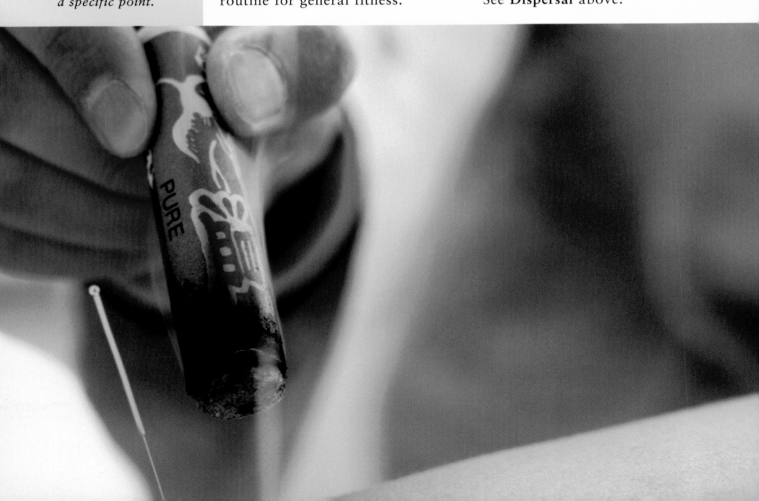

## SHEN

A Japanese word referring to the spirit or the mind. In TCM, Ki, Jing and Shen are known as "the Three Treasures". Shen provides the energy allowing us to think and to rationalise.

## TAN DEN

The **Tan Den** , also known as "the sea of Ki", is located in the abdomen, about a couple of inches beneath the navel. This is an important energetic point, corresponding to the sacral chakra, and is the body's centre of gravity.

## TCM

Traditional Chinese Medicine.

## THIRD EYE

Also known as the brow chakra, the Third Eye is located between the eyebrows. It is believed to be the seat of psychic energy and clairvoyance.

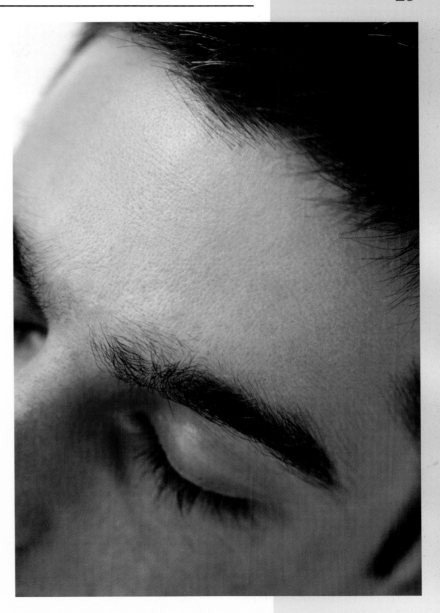

## TONIFICATION

A type of Shiatsu technique, designed to stimulate the energy level in an area.

## TRIGGER POINTS

These are similar to **ahshi** points. Pressure on trigger points causes pain in other parts of the body. Thus, working on the shoulders may refer intense pain up the neck, but will help to relax the muscles neck and shoulder muscles.

*Above: the Third Eye is located between the eyebrows.*

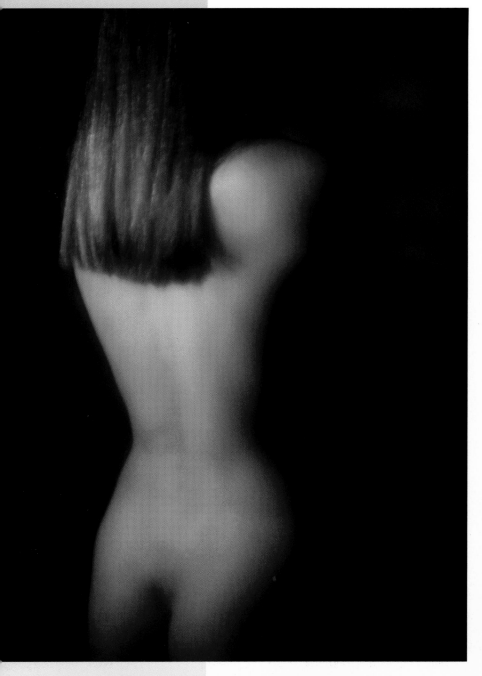

*Above: the Triple Heater is the body's main source of protection.*

## TRIPLE HEATER

The **Triple Heater** relates closely to the fluids in the body. It is also the body's main source of protection.

## TSUBO

**Tsubo** is the Japanese name for a pressure point. These are located along the meridians and correspond to certain acupuncture points. Pressure on a tsubo influences the energy flow through the meridian.

## YIN/YANG

**Yin/Yang** forms the basis of Oriental medicine. Yin and Yang are the beginning and the end, life and death. The two qualities are linked. For example, Yin is relaxed, Yang is active, but activity always ends with relaxation and relaxation, in turn, leads to more action.

## ZANG ORGANS

Usually known as Yang organs, **Zang organs** are used for storing energy. See also **Fu organs**.

## ZEN

This is a form of Buddhism, particularly popular in Japan. The spiritual approach of **Zen** forms part of Zen Shiatsu, a style developed by Shizuto Masunaga. TCM ideas are also incorporated in this style.

# HOW DOES SHIATSU WORK?

The simplest possible explanation of how Shiatsu works is to say that it uses the application of pressure on certain points in the body in order to stimulate and balance the life force. However, this reply rather begs the question, and the reader is justified in demanding, "Which pressure points?", "What is the life force?" and so on.

## TRADITIONAL CHINESE MEDICINE (TCM)

TCM is based on the principle that a vital life force flows throughout our bodies. When the Japanese adopted the practice of Shiatsu, they shared this conviction – a belief that has been confirmed by 21st-century quantum physics. Indeed, it is now known that everything we see, feel, touch or think is a manifestation of this vital energy. It is present in many different forms – in material objects such as rocks, earth, trees and, of course, human beings, as well as intangible forces. More than 2000 years ago, the Japanese called this vital force Ki and Shiatsu practitioners still use the term. In China, it is known as chi, in India it is called prana, and Native Americans refer to orenda.

*Below: energy manifests itself in many different forms – for example, material objects such as rocks, earth and trees.*

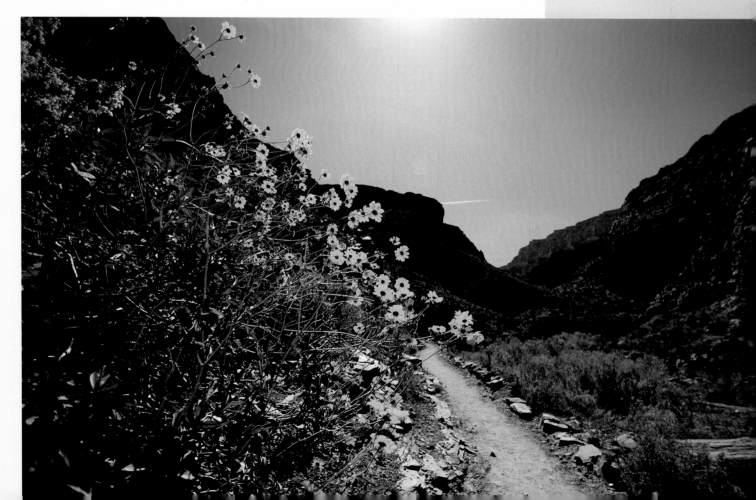

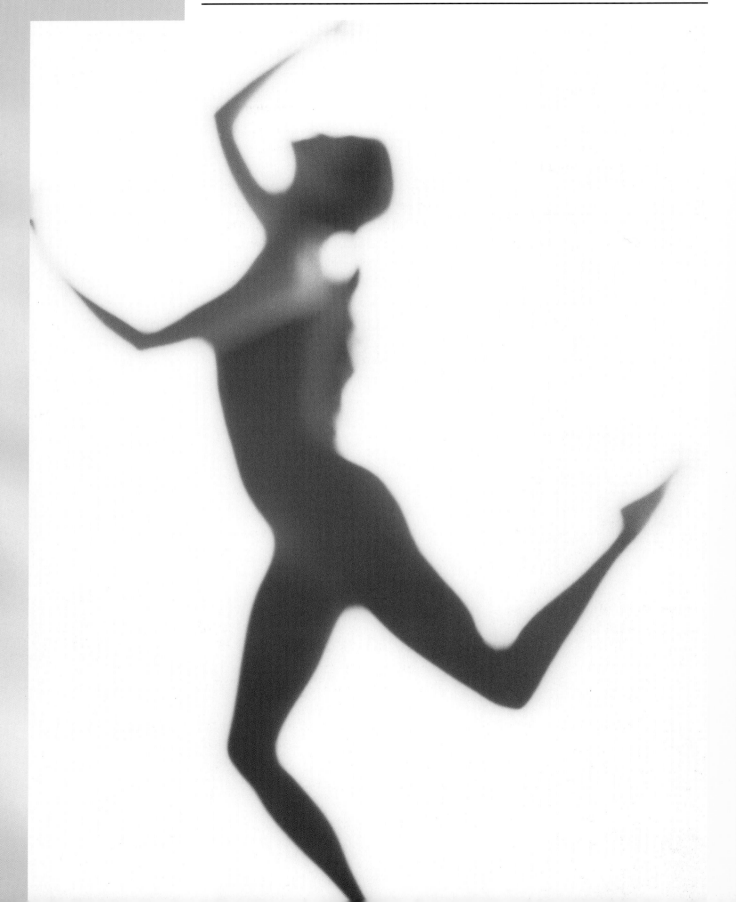

# KI – THE LIFE FORCE

Without the essential flow of Ki throughout out bodies, we would literally cease to exist. If there is a blockage to the flow of Ki in your body, you will probably become physically or emotionally ill.

## WHAT KI DOES

*It controls every type of movement, physical or mental.*

*It protects the physical body from infection, cold, heat, etc.*

*It regulates the temperature of the body.*

*It changes our food intake into the nourishment required for health.*

## EXPERIMENT WITH KI

Perhaps it is difficult to believe that such a powerful and mysterious energy can be surging through your body without you being aware of it. You may be interested in conducting a small experiment to convince you of its existence. This is a very simple procedure.

*Stand upright, feet apart, and stretch your arms up above your head.*

*Now briskly rub your palms together until they tingle with warmth. Repeat this friction on the back of your hands, the forearms and the wrists.*

*Next, drop your arms so that they hang down the sides of the body and shake them vigorously.*

*Repeat this whole procedure two or three times. Now, stretch out your hands in front of your body and notice the pleasant warm sensation. Return your arms to your sides. Take a deep breath and, as you slowly exhale, RELAX.*

Repeat this entire routine several times. Then extend your hands in front of you, palms facing, with a distance of about 12 inches (30 cm) between them. Slowly bring the palms closer together. As the space decreases, you can expect to experience a feeling of warmth and vibration between your hands. You will then know that your experiment has been successful – you can actually feel the flow of Ki between your hands.

Not only does this valuable exercise increase your awareness of Ki, it also stimulates the flow of the life force throughout your body. As with all other procedures, you will need to practise this routine until it becomes natural to you. Gradually your awareness of Ki will become stronger and you will be able to experience it more easily.

*Far left: Ki controls every type of movement, physical or mental.*

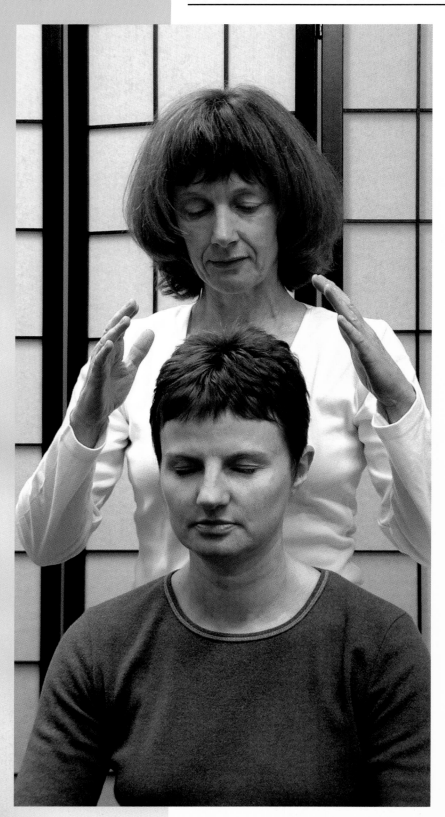

## SENSING KI IN OTHER PEOPLE

This experiment enables you to feel the flow of Ki in the aura of another person.

Ask your friend to sit upright on an ordinary dining chair. Then repeat the procedure outlined in the first exercise but, instead of having your two hands stretched out in front of you, allow one to hover about 12 inches (30 cm) above the seated person's head.

Persevere with this, moving your hand around, until you feel the tingling and warmth between your hand and your friend's head. Once this point has been reached, you can experiment further by moving your hand round the person's head and shoulders.

The flow of Ki you experience at this time comes from the etheric aura of the other person.

This exercise is particularly valuable in that it will stimulate the flow of Ki in your own body and that of your partner.

### KI BLOCKAGES

If the flow of energy becomes blocked, you will experience restrictions in the areas involved and this can lead to illness. This applies to spiritual, mental and emotional levels, as well as to the physical level. When Ki is flowing smoothly throughout the material body, other levels will also be balanced. When blockages occur, a Shiatsu practitioner can feel the imbalances and clear them by the use of stretching or pressure, in the same way that an acupuncturist uses needles.

### HOW IS IMBALANCE CAUSED?

It is safe to say that there is seldom one solitary reason for any imbalance of Ki. Shiatsu is an holistic treatment, dealing with the whole person. A practitioner knows that imbalance is usually caused by a combination of mind/body/spirit disturbances – a theory that has also become widely accepted by orthodox medicine over recent years.

Imbalances can be caused – for example – by intense anger (which will affect the liver), or by a change in the weather. For example, heavy thundery weather may give you a crashing headache.

### THREE TYPES OF KI

Traditionally, there are three types of Ki within the body.

*Grain Ki comes from the food we eat.*

*Air Ki is obtained from the air we breathe.*

*Original (or pre-natal) Ki is derived from our genetic inheritance.*

Blood is considered to be a material manifestation of Ki, designed to nourish the body's tissues.

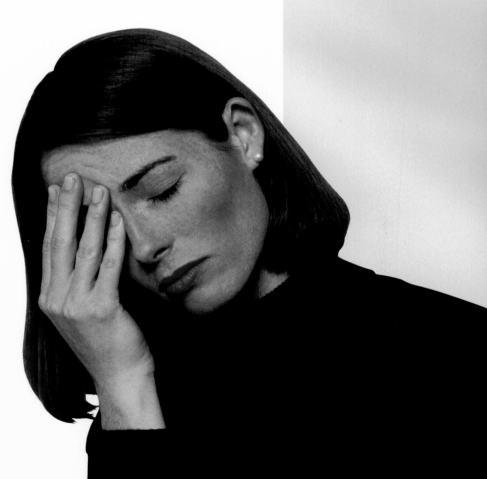

*Far left: sensing the Ki in other people is particularly valuable in that it will stimulate the flow of Ki in your own body and that of your partner.*

*Below: imbalances of Ki can be caused by intense anger or a change in the weather. For example, heavy thundery weather may give you a crashing headache.*

## KI AND THE MERIDIANS

Ki flows throughout the body in a series of connected pathways called meridians. Each of the 12 meridians is named after the organ with which it connects. There are other channels deeper within the body, but only two of these – known as the Governing Vessel and the Conception Vessel – can be used in Shiatsu treatment.

*Below: Ki flows throughout the body in a series of connected pathways called meridians.*

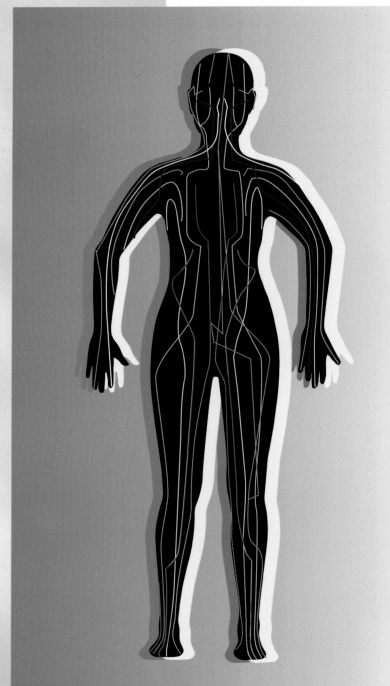

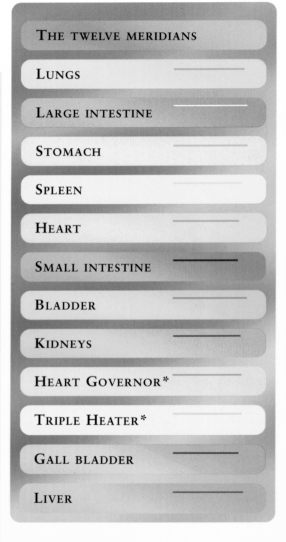

| THE TWELVE MERIDIANS |
| --- |
| LUNGS |
| LARGE INTESTINE |
| STOMACH |
| SPLEEN |
| HEART |
| SMALL INTESTINE |
| BLADDER |
| KIDNEYS |
| HEART GOVERNOR* |
| TRIPLE HEATER* |
| GALL BLADDER |
| LIVER |

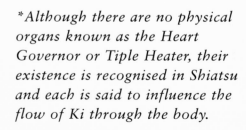

*\*Although there are no physical organs known as the Heart Governor or Tiple Heater, their existence is recognised in Shiatsu and each is said to influence the flow of Ki through the body.*

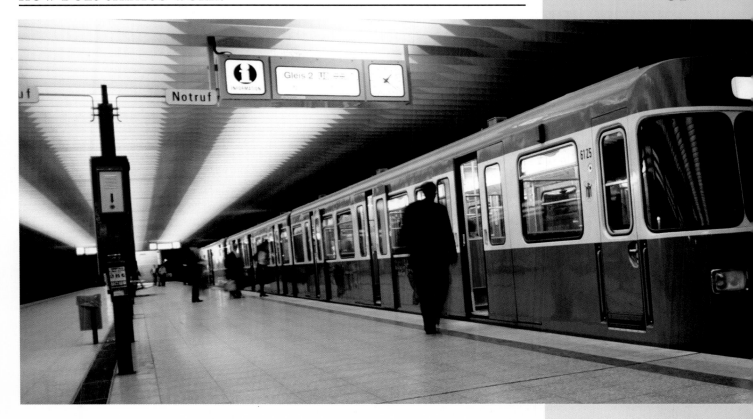

Ki's passage through the body can be likened to that of an underground train, running from one meridian ("station") to the next in a kind of loop. Thus, Ki can pass from one meridian to another via a channel ("tunnel") that links each meridian to two others.

Traditionally, the organs of the body are said to have a dual function – one physical and the other energetic (i.e. concerned with the use of energy.) They are also split into two groups – known as Yin organs (for energy storage) and Yang organs (for producing energy.)

| YIN ORGANS | YANG ORGANS |
| --- | --- |
| Lungs | Large intestine |
| Spleen | Stomach |
| Heart | Small intestine |
| Kidneys | Bladder |
| Heart Governor | Triple Heater |
| Liver | Gall bladder |

*Above: Ki's passage through the body can be likened to that of an underground train, running from one meridian ("station") to the next in a kind of loop.*

### FUNCTIONS OF THE ORGANS

**Lungs** absorb Ki from the air and ensure mental alertness.

**Large intestine** absorbs fluids, and encourages self-confidence.

**Spleen** controls digestion, and is concerned with concentration and analytical thought.

**Stomach** affects intake of nourishment and encourages harmonious feelings.

**Heart** controls blood vessels and circulation, affects emotions and memory.

**Small intestine** controls assimilation of food, and affects ability to make decisions.

**Kidneys** produce basic energy for other organs, and affect willpower and vitality.

**Bladder** stores waste fluids, affects courage and strength of mind.

**Heart Governor** protects the heart and affects relationships.

**Triple Heater** assists flow of Ki and helps social interaction.

**Liver** assists detoxification and promotes emotional calm.

**Gall bladder** controls storage/distribution of bile and encourages creativity.

### PRESSURE POINTS

Shiatsu treatment aims to affect the flow of Ki by applying pressure to certain points along the meridians. These points are known as tsubos.

But how do you know where they are? It's really quite simple and, with practice, you will soon be able to find any particular pressure point you wish. They are located in the little hollows between the bones and the muscles or near nerves – once you begin looking for them, you will be surprised at how many of these small depressions exist.

*Below: Shiatsu treatment aims to affect the flow of Ki by applying pressure to certain points along the meridians. These points are known as tsubos.*

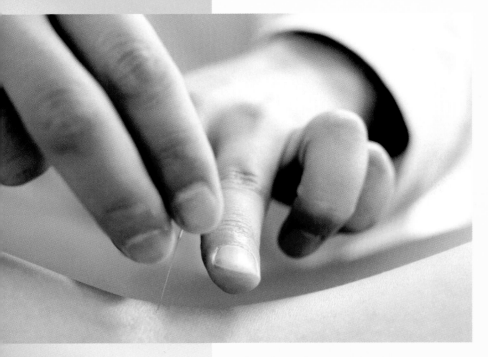

Ki circulates continuously throughout the body, but there are times when it reaches a peak in different meridians and organs. This theory is known as the Chinese Clock Cycle.

Obviously, it is not always possible to treat a certain organ or meridian at the "right" time – that is, the time at which Ki is at maximum strength in the relevant part of the body. Even so, because each meridian is associated with a particular two-hour period, the system does allow for the consideration of individual strengths and weaknesses.

Some practitioners use the Chinese Clock Cycle in a slightly different way. Instead of trying to apply treatment at the time Ki is at its peak, they take note of the time of day when symptoms appear to enable them to make an accurate diagnosis.

This Cycle theory, too, can be particularly valuable in self-treatment – for example, if your vitality seems to slump after lunch, this could indicate that the small intestine meridian needs a boost between the hours of 1 p.m. and 3 p.m.

## THE HEART GOVERNOR

Like the heart meridian, the Heart Governor is concerned with the circulation of blood throughout the body. As we have already stated, there is no organ known by this name though it is sometimes identified as the pericardium. The Heart Governor is connected with the heart and all its functions, physical and emotional.

## THE TRIPLE HEATER

The Triple Heater works closely with the Heart Governor and facilitates the passage of Ki around the body. It regulates body temperature and also acts in a protective capacity since it covers the immune system.

*Below: the chinese clock cycle.*

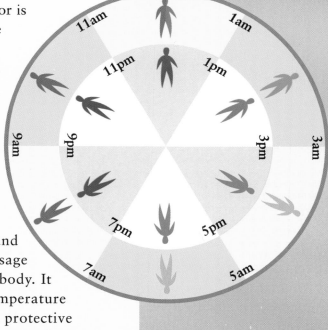

| MERIDIAN KI AT MAXIMUM FLOW | | | |
|---|---|---|---|
| Liver | 1a.m. to 3a.m. | Small intestine | 1p.m. to 3p.m. |
| Lungs | 3a.m. to 5a.m. | Bladder | 3p.m. to 5p.m. |
| Large intestine | 5a.m. to 7a.m. | Kidneys | 5p.m. to 7p.m. |
| Stomach | 7a.m. to 9a.m. | Heart Governor | 7p.m.to 9p.m. |
| Spleen | 9a.m. to 11a.m. | Triple Heater | 9p.m. to 11p.m. |
| Heart | 11a.m. to 1p.m. | Gall bladder | 11p.m. to 1a.m. |

# YIN AND YANG

Most people recognise the distinctive black and white Yin and Yang symbol, even if they have no idea what it means.

Yin and Yang are the two complementary aspects of Ki. According to Huang Ti, the famous Chinese Yellow Emperor, Yin/Yang is the basic principle of everything that is. There can be no life without death, no heat without cold, no night without day, no negative without positive and so on.

## LIFE FORCE OF THE UNIVERSE

Ki is the vital life force of the entire Universe. Yin and Yang are two aspects of that force. Both are found in different proportions – not only in all material or physical objects, but also in intangible qualities like rest and activity, cold and warmth, slow and fast.

No single quality or object is completely Yin or Yang, but everything in the Universe possesses a proportion of both, being predominantly Yin or predominantly Yang.

## TRANSFORMATION

Yin and Yang are invariably interconnected and each has the ability to transform the other. For example, Water is considered to be Yin. Fire (which is Yang) transforms water into steam, which is also Yang. Cold (which is Yin) transforms the steam (Yang) back into water – which is Yin. Despite this constant state of transformation between Yin and Yang, the end result is always one of balance.

## YIN/YANG IN THE BODY

The meridians that act as channels for the flow of Ki are themselves divided between Yin and Yang. Yang meridians are associated with the more solid organs like the heart, kidneys and spleen. These

*Below: Yin and Yang are invariably interconnected and each has the ability to transform the other. For example, Water is considered to be Yin. Fire (which is Yang) transforms water into steam, which is also Yang.*

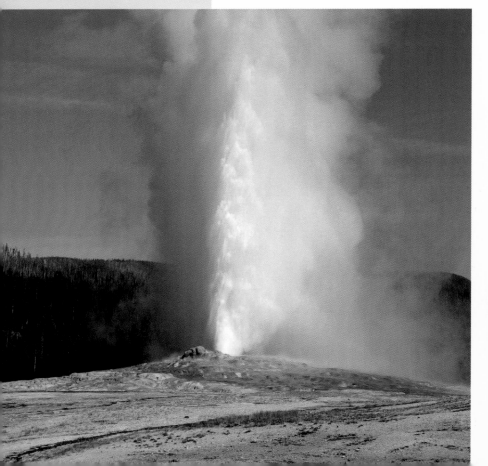

channels are located down the back of the body and the outer edges of the limbs. Yin meridians serve what are termed "hollow organs" – stomach, small intestine and bladder – which are found in the front of the body.

## Yin organs   Yang organs

| | |
|---|---|
| *Large intestine* | *Lungs* |
| *Small intestine* | *Heart* |
| *Stomach* | *Spleen* |
| *Bladder* | *Kidneys* |
| *Triple Heater* | *Heart* |
| | *Governor* |
| *Gall bladder* | *Liver* |

In ancient China, the word Yin meant "dark side of the mountain" and Yang applied to the bright, sunny side. Similarly, the Yang side of the body is the back, the side that is usually in the sun. The Yin side – the one more likely to be in shadow – is the front.

Yin is feminine, Yang is masculine. Yin energy is placid and stable and flows upwards. Yang energy is vigorous and transforming and flows downwards. Yin represents earth, the moon, water, darkness. Yang typifies heaven, the sun, heat and light.

The Yin/Yang principle even applies to food. Thus – milk, honey, sugar, fruit juice, vegetables and fruit are defined as Yin, but poultry, fish, meat, salt, cheese and eggs are Yang.

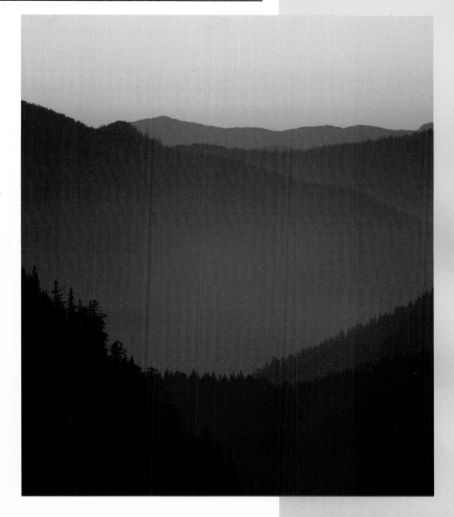

*Above: Yin means "darks side of the mountain"; Yang applies to the bright, sunny side.*

## Are you Yin or Yang?

The Yin/Yang symbol clearly shows that the two qualities together produce a perfect balance. Moreover, there is within each a certain part of the other – as indicated by the white dot on the black section and the black dot on the white.

A young woman, though basically feminine and therefore predominantly Yin, will certainly have more Yang traits than an old woman. As a man reaches a great age, his Yang traits will probably be superseded by Yin qualities. Psychologists agree that even the most feminine of women will sometimes reveal a certain masculine aspect to her nature, just as every "Jack the lad" undoubtedly has a feminine side.

Using the Yin/Yang theory, it is possible to make a fairly accurate assessment of the people you meet. Yin people (male or female) tend to be introverted and given to intellectual pursuits. Yang people are more extrovert and prefer physical activities.

Yin people are likely to be lethargic, to feel the cold, to be permanently sleepy. Yang people tend to be over-active, to suffer from insomnia, and to feel the heat.

## Yin/Yang and Shiatsu

It is worthwhile to decide whether you yourself are predominantly a Yin or Yang type of person, so that you will more clearly understand the working of Shiatsu. Most practitioners use the theory to ascertain what form of treatment is most likely to benefit a client. Linked to the Five Elements system, the Yin/Yang theory illustrates exactly how energy works.

### Yin/Yang qualities

| YIN | YANG |
| --- | --- |
| Winter | Summer |
| Day | Night |
| Earth | Heaven |
| Dark | Light |
| Cold | Heat |
| Down | Up |
| Inner | Outer |
| Passive | Active |
| Moon | Sun |
| Water | Fire |
| Soft | Hard |
| Slow | Quick |
| Mental | Physical |
| North | South |
| Female | Male |

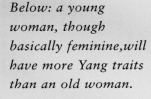

*Below: a young woman, though basically feminine, will have more Yang traits than an old woman.*

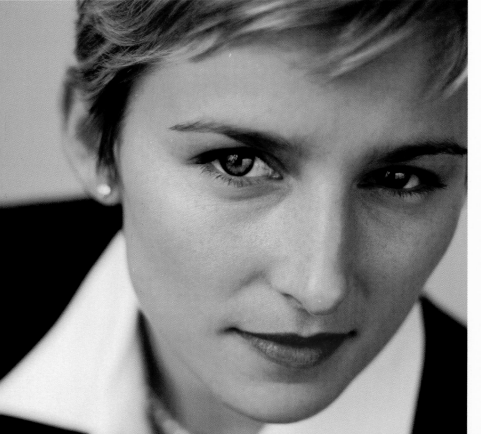

# THE FIVE ELEMENTS

The theory of the Five Elements appears in many aspects of Oriental medicine and culture, and offers a more detailed explanation of exactly how energy works. Traditionally, each element is thought to possess various attributes and to control different aspects of the body and the emotions.

## WHAT ARE THE FIVE ELEMENTS?

The Five Elements are defined as wood, fire, earth, metal and water. Each Element is considered to create the next in what is called the Creative (or Shen) Cycle. Thus:

- *Wood creates fire;*
- *Fire (ashes) enriches earth;*
- *Earth contains metal;*
- *Metal condenses water;*
- *Water feeds wood.*

Conversely, alternate Elements are said to exert a controlling influence on each other in what is known as the Control (or Ko) Cycle:

- *Fire melts metal;*
- *Metal cuts wood;*
- *Wood penetrates earth;*
- *Earth limits the flow of water;*
- *Water extinguishes fire.*

## CORRESPONDENCES

As stated earlier, the elements are traditionally associated with different aspects of the body and the emotions. Because the elements and the organs or body parts share similar energies they are known as "correspondences":

- *Wood – the liver and the gall bladder*
- *Fire – the heart and the small intestine*
- *Earth – the spleen and the stomach*
- *Metal – the lungs and the large intestine*
- *Water – the kidneys and the bladder*

*Below: the five elements and their relationships in the creative cycle and the control cyle.*

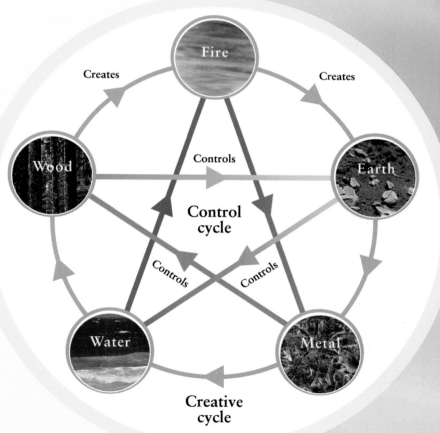

### THE SEASONS

The changing seasons, too, offer perfect examples of how one energy phase flows smoothly into the next.

**Spring** reflects **wood** energy – everything begins to grow, a surge of activity starts the year.

**Summer** corresponds to the energy of **fire** – the whole of nature is in full bloom and flourishing.

**Late summer** is the time when everything is ripening and reflects the mellow **earth** energy.

**Autumn** reflects **metal** energy, when everything gradually returns to the earth.

**Winter** is the time of cold, stillness and silence, reflecting the energy of **water**.

In fact, the seasons provide a clear illustration of the ongoing cycle of energy between Yin and Yang. This is also reflected in the relationship between the elements and their emotional correspondences.

*Below: the changing seasons offer perfect examples of how one energy phase flows smoothly into the next.*

### COLOURS

And finally, each of the Five Elements is identified by a particular colour.

- *Wood – green*
- *Fire – red*
- *Earth – yellow*
- *Metal – white*
- *Water – blue/black*

### WHICH ELEMENT TYPE ARE YOU?

Everything in nature shares in the energies of the Five Elements and human beings are no exception. Indeed, most Shiatsu practitioners use the Five Element theory as a sound diagnostic tool when treating their clients. You can also use it for deciding why your friends and family act as they do – or, for that matter, why you seem to be such a mass of contradictions.

### WOOD PEOPLE

Wood people tend to be tall and muscular, often having dark colouring. They are creative and well organised; the sort of people who like to be in charge and don't take kindly to subordinate positions. They can be noisy, particularly when angry, and sometimes display a childish attitude when crossed.

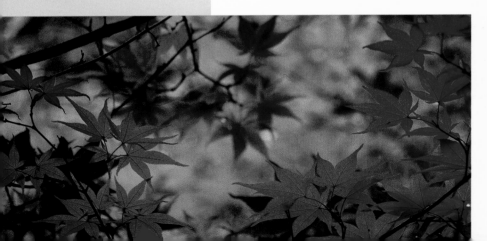

## TABLE OF GENERAL CORRESPONDANCE

| ELEMENT | SEASON | BODY PARTS | COLOUR |
|---------|--------|-----------|--------|
| Wood | Spring | Liver/gall bladder | Green |
| Fire | Summer | Heart/small intestine | Red |
| Earth | Late Summer | Spleen/stomach | Yellow |
| Metal | Fall | Lungs/large intestine | White |
| Water | Winter | Kidneys/bladder | Black/blue |

### FIRE PEOPLE

Fire people often have a ruddy complexion and may have red hair. They have a fairly small physique and usually move quickly and gracefully. Their emotions run close to the surface and they don't hesitate to express them. When they're happy, their laughter can be quite infectious. If they're sad, they can show an almost adolescent petulance. But they do have a more serious side to their nature and may be interested in spiritual matters.

### EARTH PEOPLE

Earth people sometimes have a weight problem and tend to shuffle, rather than walk briskly.

They are often sallow or olive-skinned. These are the kind of friends you need when you're in trouble, because they will be full of ideas for solving your problems. They're extremely supportive, practical and compassionate, but can be somewhat opinionated.

### METAL PEOPLE

Metal people are often good looking, tall and broad shouldered. They are well-mannered but extremely reserved, with a strong sense of personal pride. They're not the most cheerful people to have around and can sometimes, for no apparent reason, burst into floods of tears. On the whole, they're well-balanced and sensible and adopt a practical approach to most aspects of life.

### WATER PEOPLE

Water people are tall and strong and often have beautiful hair. They move easily and gracefully. They are extremely adaptable and ambitious, though there is often a lazy streak in their make-up. These people can be stubborn, and will often be fearful in situations they don't understand. "Still waters run deep" is a phrase that is often used to describe this type of person.

*Below: fire people often have a ruddy complexion and may have red hair.*

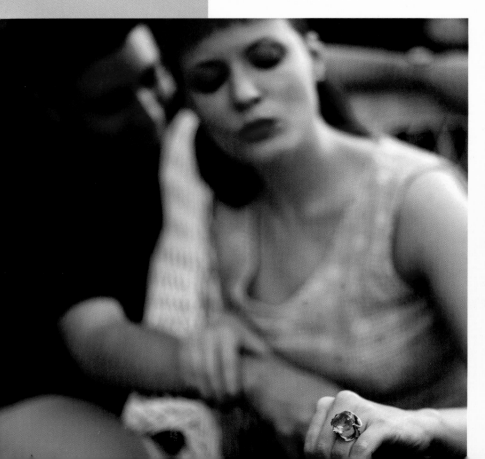

Identifying and balancing the distortions that can occur in the
meridians is an integral part of the Zen Shiatsu system and is known
as the Kyo-Jitsu theory. Kyo means empty, depleted or lacking in energy.
Jitsu has the opposite meaning – full, blocked or over-active.

Thus if a particular channel is
lacking in Ki it is defined as Kyo –
the meridian is empty or deficient
in energy. This produces a state of
hyper-activity (Jitsu) elsewhere in
that channel in an attempt to
restore the necessary balance.

Like Yin and Yang, Kyo and Jitsu
are inextricably linked. One does
not exist without the other. As an
example, if you are hungry (i.e.
empty and therefore in a Kyo
state), you will set about getting
some food. The energy expended
in this way is Jitsu – and will
restore a comfortable balance.
Your hunger will be assuaged and
the flow of Ki will be restored.

Kyo and Jitsu conditions are in a
state of constant fluctuation. The
practitioner's job is to find the
cause for any disharmony and to
put it right.

## LOCATING PROBLEM AREAS

Kyo's nature is Yin and the
affected areas are difficult to find.
They feel resistant and empty to
the touch. Jitsu is Yang in nature.
The points feel active and bouncy,
protruding from the surface.

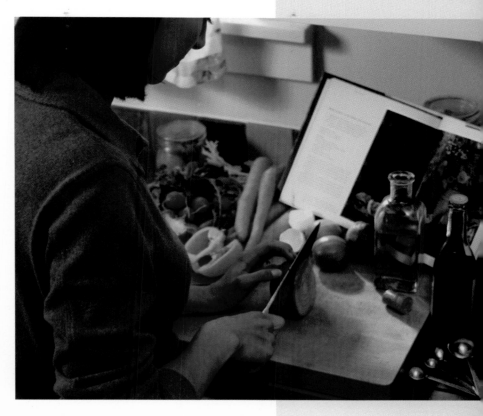

Because Kyo is a passive (Yin)
state, it is unlikely to create
symptoms, but the Jitsu (Yang)
reaction it produces can often
cause tension or pain in the related
pressure point. A professional
Shiatsu practitioner will have no
difficulty in locating the meridian
most lacking in Ki (Kyo) or the
one that is over-active (Jitsu). He
will then restore the balance
between the two channels,
whereupon all other meridians will
harmonise themselves.

*Above: if you are
hungry you will set
about getting some
food. The energy
expended in this way
is Jitsu – and will
restore a comfortable
balance.*

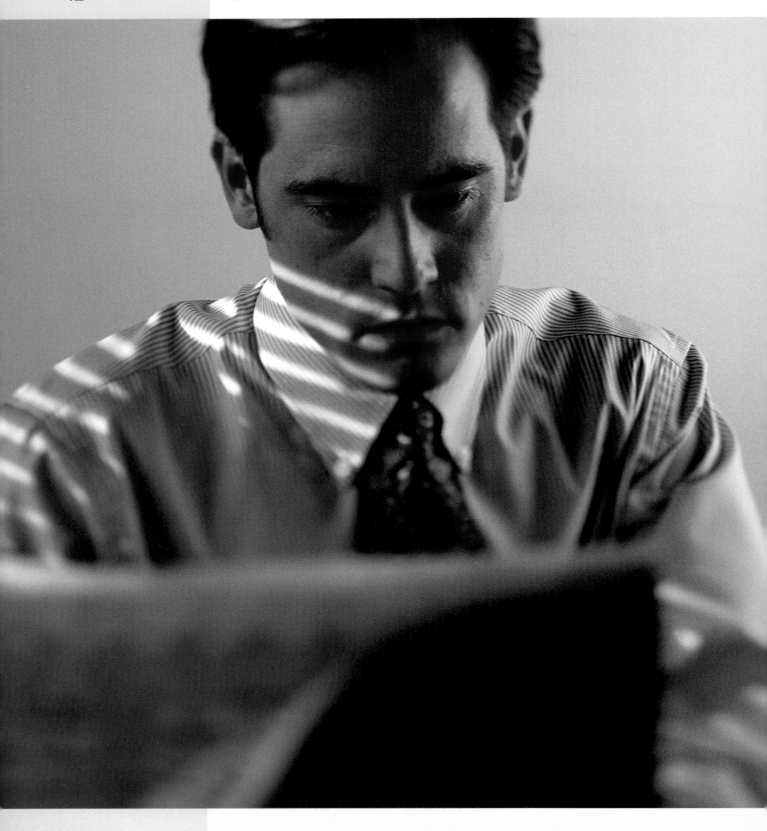

As you learn more about Shiatsu, you will realise that this is not only a form of bodywork or exercise. It is an holistic discipline that involves every aspect of your life – body, mind and spirit. You will gradually recognise the flow of Ki throughout your body – and this very awareness will serve to increase the life energy. Not only will this enhance your physical being, but your mind, emotions and spirit, too.

Your constant awareness of the power of Ki will also alter many of your ideas about other people, whether they are family, friends of long standing, casual acquaintances or tradespeople. As the theories of Yin and Yang and the Five Elements become an integral part of your awareness, you will discover that you even read a newspaper with different eyes. Because you now see everything in terms of energy, you will be able to interpret events – whether they are in your own home town or in far distant countries – from a totally different viewpoint.

with other people. When your irritable, demanding boss suddenly appears to become good-natured and considerate, it could mean that he has seen the error of his ways. The apparent change is more likely to be due to the fact that your own attitude towards him has altered. Other people may still find him tetchy and trying, but your understanding of the working of Ki has given you a different perspective. The fact is that the poor man has an excess of Yang and the wood element – hence his unfortunate attitude.

*Far left: as the theories of Yin and Yang and the Five Elements become an integral part of your awareness, you will discover that you even read a newspaper with different eyes.*

*Below: other people may still find a demanding boss tetchy and trying, but your understanding of the working of Ki will give you a different perspective.*

## TAKING CONTROL

The hurly burly of 21st-century living must surely be the root cause for many of the illnesses and weaknesses that beset us. The good news is that Shiatsu, properly used, can enable you to control stress and tension and restore a feeling of balance to your life.

Once you develop the Shiatsu habit, you will find that you are more relaxed in every way and this is sure to affect your relationships

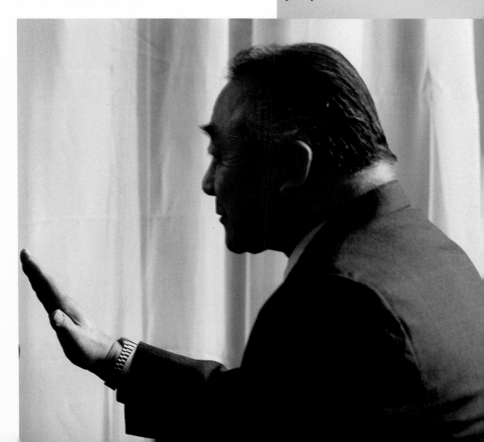

Below: the position
known as the seiza, is
ideal, but can be
difficult for some
people.

Similarly, when you feel unaccountably frustrated or depressed, you will be able to employ your knowledge to give yourself a brief Shiatsu treatment. However, since prevention is always better than cure, you will be well advised to spend some time each day on doing the physical and mental exercises listed below.

Don't feel guilty if at first you can spend only 10 minutes on these exercises. The chances are that you will find them so beneficial that you will suddenly discover that you can spare half an hour, after all. And if things don't work out that way, just accept that 10 minutes' exercise is better than no exercise at all.

## DEVELOPING THE HARA

Hara is the Japanese word for the abdomen which Oriental medicine considers to be the seat of the life force. This is also the body's centre of gravity and the site of the Tan Den, one of the major energy centres (or chakras) in the body. It is located about two inches below your navel. The object of this first exercise is to focus your attention on the Tan Den. An ability to do this at will is sure to enhance greatly your tranquillity and powers of concentration and "centre" your emotions.

## FOCUSING ON THE TAN DEN

Sit in a comfortable position on the floor. The position shown in the illustration, known as the seiza, is ideal, but can be difficult for some people. You may find it easier to sit with crossed legs. It is important to be comfortable because this exercise demands complete relaxation.

Take time to ensure that every part of your body is soft and totally at ease. This in itself may be difficult if you are not accustomed to relaxation, but persevere. Be careful not to tense your muscles in a desperate attempt to relax them. Simply quieten your mind and allow your body to slump.

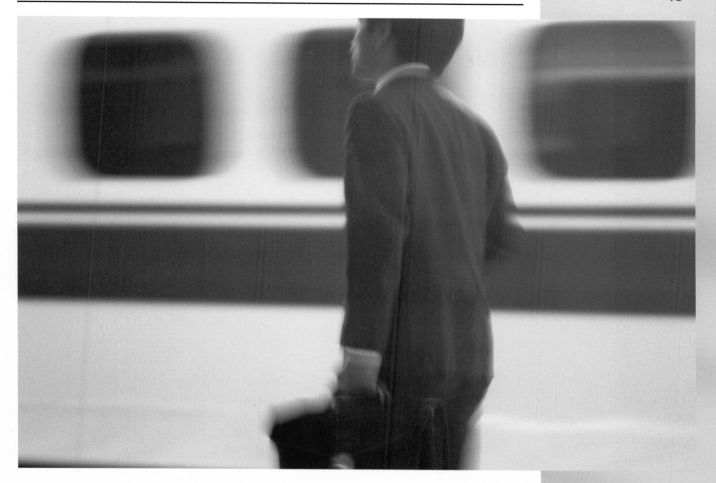

When your whole body is relaxed, sit up as straight as possible – again, without tension – with your palms placed gently on the lower abdomen. Begin breathing deeply and rhythmically into the Tan Den. As you breathe in through your nose, allow your belly to swell out. When you breathe out, your stomach muscles will contract. Continue to breathe in this way for a few minutes, concentrating on the breath itself.

Next, shift your concentration to the hara and feel the Ki within it.

Visualise energy flowing into the hara with every breath you take. Try to do this exercise for about five minutes every day. In time you will find that you can become aware of the hara and its energy whenever you wish – waiting for a bus or at the supermarket check-out, taking a shower or travelling to work. It is a valuable method of enhancing your Ki awareness and entering into a relaxed state.

*Above: in time you will find that you can become aware of the hara and its energy whenever you wish - even in the hustle of travelling to work.*

# THE HUMAN AURA.

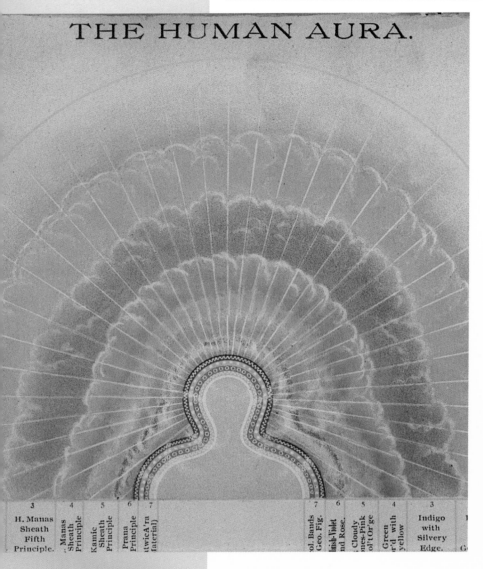

| 3 | 4 | 5 | 6 | 7 | | 7 | 6 | 5 | 4 | 3 | |
|---|---|---|---|---|---|---|---|---|---|---|---|
| H. Manas Sheath Fifth Principle. | Manas Sheath Principle | Kamic Sheath Principle | Prana Principle | itwicA'ra laterial) | | ol. Bands Geo. Fig. | nish-Violet nd Rose. | Cloudy nes-Pink ol'tOr'ge | Green r'd with yellow | Indigo with Silvery Edge. | G. |

*Above: the radiant coloured aura, seen by clairvoyants; a lithograph from Marquès 'The Human Aura' 1896.*

## AURAS

It is now generally acknowledged that Ki affects not only the physical body but the auras (or energy fields) that surround it.

First there is the **etheric body** which is the most dense of the auras and is closely connected with the physical body. The next aura – the **astral body** – is wider than the etheric and is much affected by personal feelings. A clairvoyant is able to see this aura and can tell, from the way it changes shape and colour, exactly how you are feeling. The mental body comes next. This, too, can be seen by a clairvoyant, and is much concerned with your thought processes and intellect.

These first three auras (counted from the body outwards) comprise your personality. The last aura has several names – the soul, the higher self, and the **causal body** are but three. Reincarnationists believe that it is this last aura that continues to develop after death and goes on to adopt another body and personality.

### KI AND THE AURAS

As your wisdom and understanding increase, throughout your life, the different auras are used and energy passes from one layer to another. Obviously, this means that any changes in your physical state will be reflected in the auras and will affect the flow of Ki.

# THE CHAKRAS

As previously stated, the Tan Den is one of the chakras (energy centres) found in the body. There are seven in all, positioned along the spiritual channel running from the crown of the head to the base of the torso.

These areas are activated as a person develops, physically and emotionally. There is also a transfer of energy between the auras and the chakras.

The **crown chakra** is located on the top of the head and it is concerned with the pineal gland. It also affects your spiritual development.

The **brow chakra**, as its name suggests, is found between and behind the eyebrows. It is also known as the Third Eye. It is linked with the pituitary gland, controlling the nose, the nervous system, and the left eye. Focusing on the brow chakra will develop insight, intuitive faculties and psychic ability.

The **throat chakra** is concerned with the thyroid gland and therefore the metabolism of your body. It also controls the lymphatic system and affects your self-expression, your creative powers and communication.

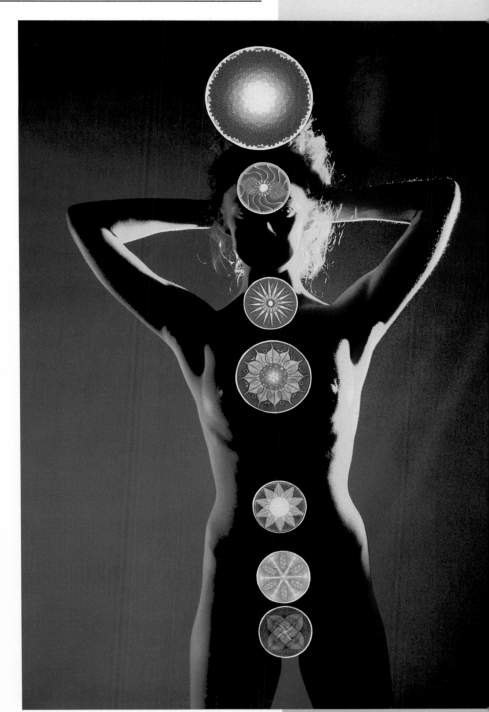

*Above: the seven chakras distributed over the body*

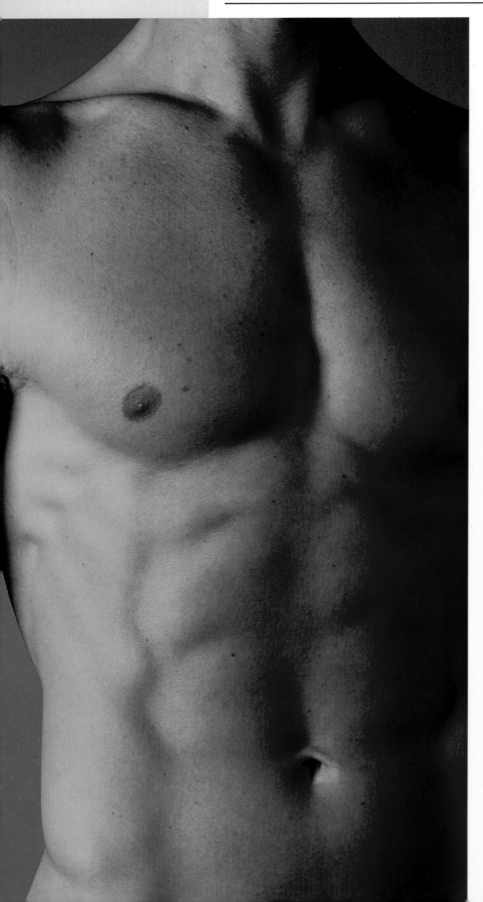

The **heart chakra** is found in the middle of the upper chest and governs the thymus gland. It controls the heart, chest and circulation, but is particularly concerned with the emotions. Some practitioners use the heart centre in a similar way to that described above for the Tan Den. You may find it helpful to breathe into this area when you have any emotional problems.

The **solar plexus chakra** links with the pancreas and controls the liver, gall bladder, and digestive system. It also affects your ego and your emotions.

The **sacral chakra** controls the lower back and the sexual organs. It affects your physical and mental energy, your self-worth and personal relationships.

The **base chakra** is concerned with the production of adrenalin and controls the skeleton, the nervous system and the reproductive system. It is linked with your ability to express your emotions.

# MEDITATION

In Shiatsu, exercises to calm the mind are just as important as physical exercises. The traditional way to do this is by meditation.

Some people find this difficult, probably because they are under the mistaken impression that meditating means emptying the mind or thinking about nothing. In fact, there is a wide variety of meditation techniques, most of which involve breathing exercises and visualisation. The meditation detailed below is very simple and, because it is short, is particularly suitable if this is your first attempt. You will almost certainly find it difficult (a) to ignore the

*Far left: the heart chakra is found in the middle of the upper chest and governs the thymus gland. It controls the heart, chest and circulation, but is particularly concerned with the emotions.*

*Left: in Shiatsu, the traditional way to calm the mind is by meditation.*

"monkey chatter" in your head and (b) to maintain a state of contemplation for more than a few minutes. Don't worry about this. Instead of struggling to keep your mind fixed on the golden light, allow thoughts to drift as they will. The secret lies in not paying attention to them. Let them drift into focus and out again, then gently bring your concentration back to your meditation.

As with all aspects of Shiatsu "practice makes perfect". In time you will be able to meditate at will and enjoy the considerable benefits to be gained from this practice.

*Below: for meditation some people like to sit on a chair, some prefer to be cross-legged on the floor and others adopt the seiza position.*

## GOLDEN LIGHT MEDITATION

This exercise takes only 10 minutes but, if done correctly, will re-energise you when you are tired and replace negative thoughts with the positive variety.

As always, make yourself comfortable in any way most convenient for you. Some people like to sit on a chair, some prefer to be cross-legged on the floor and others adopt the seiza position. Try to keep your back straight, but not tense.

As already explained, breathe quietly and regularly into the hara. Close your eyes. When you feel ready, take a deep breath. As you inhale, visualise your entire body filling with Ki.

Imagine it as a beautiful golden light, flowing through the meridians until your body is completely suffused with energy. Sit quietly, breathing regularly and basking in the sensation of warmth and light. Then, as you exhale, breathe the golden light into the room.

Repeat the process as often as you wish, but remain relaxed and comfortable. If you begin to tire or tense up, it's time to stop.

This exercise can be particularly helpful when you have painful problems such as backache. Breathe the golden light into the affected area then, as you exhale, visualise the pain leaving your body.

## REGULAR ROUTINE

The exercises given in this section of the book are simple but beneficial. Try to use them every day. However, it is important that you should not feel stressed or try to perform the routines in a rush. No aspect of Shiatsu can be hurried and it is better to spend just five minutes on hara breathing than to attempt to deal with the whole sequence at top speed.

Do-In is a self-development routine traditionally used as a warm-up procedure in martial arts. It is also widely used at the beginning of Shiatsu classes.

There are many variations of this routine, some taking a great deal longer than others. We will deal with only three types of Do-In exercises, all of which can be achieved in a comparatively short time. Here again, though, it is important that you should not attempt to cram too much into the time available.

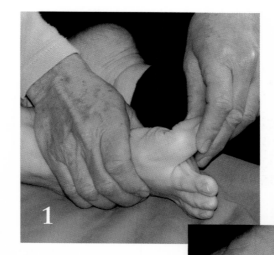

First, let's look at the most simple method of all, involving only the hands and feet.

## SHORT DO-IN

First, enjoy a good long stretch, then allow your body to slump. Next, vigorously shake your hands to disperse any remaining tension. Now you are ready for your first experience of Do-In.

*1. Sit on the floor, take hold of one big toe and pull gently, at the same time rotating it. Rotate again in the opposite direction. Do this for a few seconds, then repeat the actions on the other foot.*

*2. Hold each toe in turn, gently pressing it backwards until you feel tension in the underside. Breathe steadily and maintain the pressure for a count of 10.*

*3. Lightly clench your right fist. Support your left foot with the left hand, then roll the knuckles of your right fist all over the sole for a few seconds. Repeat the procedure on your right foot, supporting it with your right hand and using the knuckles of your left fist.*

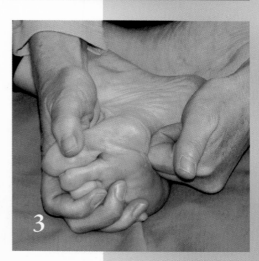

If you have difficulty in sitting on the floor, you will be able to perform the exercises equally well while sitting on your bed.

*Right: if you perform these exercises every day, you will swiftly notice increased flexibility and strength in your hands and feet.*

*Far right: the hara plays an important part in maintaining your energy flow.*

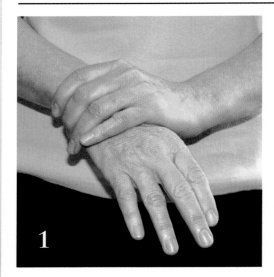

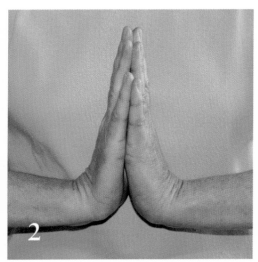

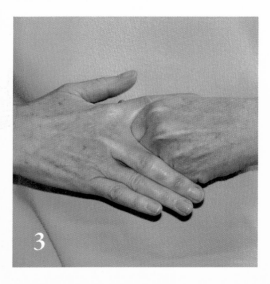

*1. Using your right hand, grip your left hand just below the wrist. Squeeze the left hand gently and slide your right hand slowly down it, working from the wrist to the fingertips.*

*2. Bring your palms together in front of your chest, fingers pointing up. Press the palms towards each other and down. You will feel pressure in the heels of your hands. Now turn the hands so that the fingers are pointing down. Press the palms together, as before, but this time inwards and upwards.*

*3. Close one hand into a fist. Push this between two of the fingers on the other hand and press down until you feel a stretch. Repeat this with all fingers and then follow the same procedure with the other hand.*

**NB:** When practising these exercises, remember always to work on both sides – left and right – equally.

If you perform these exercises every day, you will swiftly notice increased flexibility and strength in your hands and feet.

As already emphasised, the hara plays an important part in maintaining your energy flow. Exercising the abdomen area helps to keep it supple and lessens the likelihood of such problems as constipation and indigestion.

*Lie flat on your back, feet on the floor, bending your knees upwards.*

*1. Link the fingers of each hand together over the abdomen.*

*Rock the hara gently for a few minutes. You should feel your intestines moving beneath your hands.*

*If this feels comfortable, add a little more pressure before returning to the gentle movement as you finish the exercise.*

*2. With your fingers, begin to press in at the top of the hara*

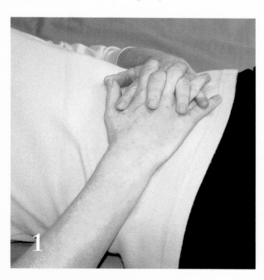

*(the solar plexus chakra). Move your fingers to the left as you inhale, then press in again as you breathe out. Some people have difficulty in synchronising this movement with the required breathing pattern. Practise it separately for a while and, quite suddenly, the idea will click!*

*3. Continue with these movements inside the ribs and all round the hara.*

*4. The final movement in hara massage is to place your interlaced hands over the Tan Den and relax for five minutes or more.*

**NB:** Resist the temptation to jump up as soon as you have completed this exercise. Relax for a few minutes until you are ready to return to the "real" world.

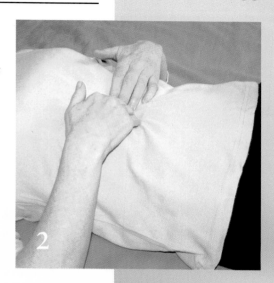

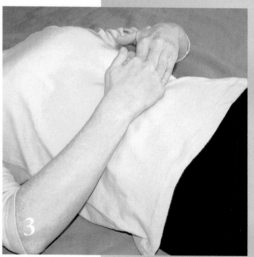

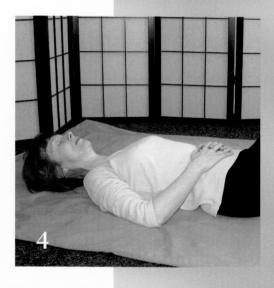

# MAKKO-HO

Shizuto Masunaga, the man who introduced Zen Shiatsu to the West, devised the Makko-ho system of exercises. These six stretches are often used at the beginning of a Shiatsu class, and they also form a set of exercises in their own right. Do them every day and your body will become noticeably more supple.

*Right: the six stretches are often used at the beginning of a Shiatsu class. The two shown here are the Governing Vessel (left) and the Conception Vessel (right) which often preceed the others.*

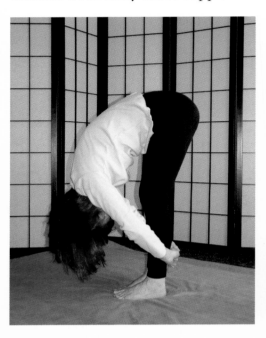 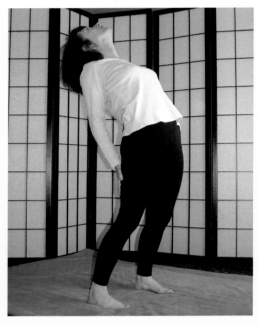

Makko-ho exercises are designed to stretch and stimulate each pair of meridians. If you are aware of a blockage in one specific organ or meridian, try the appropriate exercise as a first aid remedy. You will almost certainly notice an improvement.

### DON'T RUSH

As with all forms of exercise, it is a mistake to rush into Makko-ho. First study the illustrations and instructions carefully. Read them several times before you attempt to do any of the stretches. Don't be disheartened if, at first, you find the exercises difficult. Perfection takes practice. As your body becomes more supple, your performance will improve and you will notice that Ki is flowing more smoothly.

### BEFORE YOU BEGIN

It is not a good idea to perform these exercises when you are tired or tense or slightly stiff – as when you first get out of bed. If you plan to start each day with a Makko-ho session, you could use the first of the Do-In exercises to warm up beforehand.

Alternatively, simply stand up straight, stretch your arms up and out and breathe in. As you breathe out, lower the arms and relax. This exercise is particularly beneficial if performed in front of an open window or – weather permitting – in the open air.

## BREATHING AWARENESS

Like most Oriental therapies, Shiatsu places great emphasis on the importance of correct breathing. Learning to inhale and exhale in the right places can be difficult, but there is no need to worry about it. As with everything connected with Shiatsu, the breathing question should be considered slowly and calmly. Console yourself with the certain knowledge that you will eventually get it right – and it doesn't matter how long it takes.

Breathing awareness is a form of meditation. Practised regularly, it will help you to master the intricacies of the "right" breathing for Shiatsu. Additionally, it will give you peace of mind and help you to feel "centred".

## MEDITATING WITH MAKKO-HO

Try to undertake your Makko-ho meditation at the same time, for the same period and in the same room every day. The advice given in previous sections applies here. Ensure as far as possible that you will not be disturbed and that the room is airy but comfortably warm. If it is too warm you will be too drowsy to meditate, but if it is too cold you will be too chilly to relax.

Choose a position in which you feel comfortable and which enables you to breathe deeply and regularly. You may sit on an upright chair or cross-legged on the floor – but you are advised not to stretch out on a bed or sofa, where you are likely to fall asleep.

*Close your eyes, settle yourself comfortably and relax.*

*Breathe normally, to begin with. Then gradually make each breath slower and deeper.*

*Focus your attention on the feeling of your breath as it enters and leaves your nostrils.*

*Now turn your attention to the sound your breath makes as it enters and leaves your body. Focus on this for a few minutes.*

*Be aware that as you inhale your stomach swells, and as you exhale it contracts.*

*Remain in the meditative state for as long as you wish.*

### BREATHING PATTERNS

Breathing is an important aspect of all six stretches. Basically, the pattern is that you inhale in the first position, exhale on the stretch, and inhale as you release it.

Like the exercises themselves, this breathing pattern may take time to master. There is no need to worry about this and you should certainly not cause yourself any discomfort by struggling to fit the breathing to the exercise. Master the movements first and you will find eventually that the breathing will correspond.

### EXERCISE 1 – LUNG/LARGE INTESTINE

These channels relate to the METAL element.

*1. Standing with your feet apart, link your thumbs behind your back.*

*2. Breathing out, lean forward, keeping your arms straight out behind you.*

*3. If possible, gradually bring your arms further over your head and relax into the stretch, breathing quietly and regularly.*

*4. Exhale as you slowly straighten up.*

**Caution:** *Do not attempt the lung/large intestine stretch if you have low blood pressure or suffer from back trouble.*

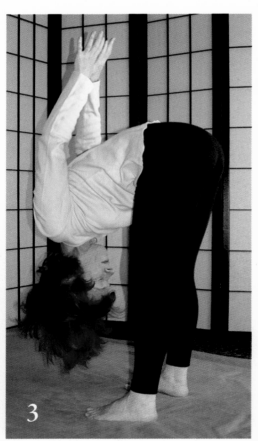

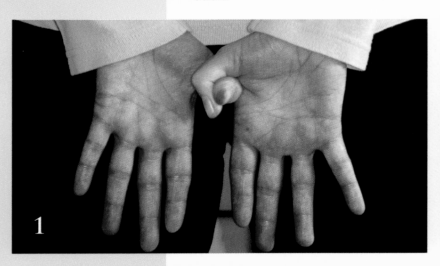

### EXERCISE 2 – STOMACH/SPLEEN

These channels relate to the EARTH element.

*1. Kneel, knees slightly parted to allow your buttocks to touch the floor. (If you cannot do this, use a small cushion to sit on.)*

*2. As you exhale, lean back and support yourself on your arms, with your hands on the floor behind you. Remain in this position, breathing gently.*

*3. If you are exceptionally supple, you may be able to stretch all the way back until you are laying on the floor with your arms stretched out above your head.*

*4. Inhale as you return to the upright position.*

**Caution:** *Always remember to remain in whichever leaning-back position is most comfortable for you. Don't try to force anything.*

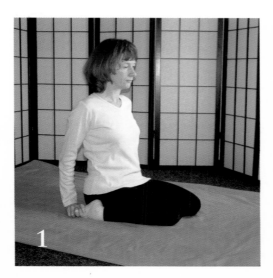

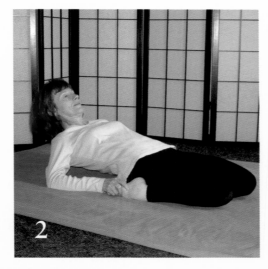

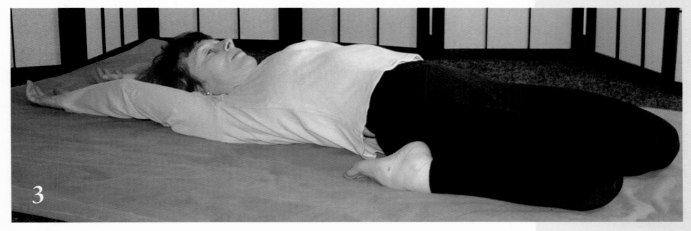

### EXERCISE 3 – HEART/SMALL INTESTINE

These meridians relate to the FIRE element.

*1. Sit on the floor with the soles of your feet together.*

*2. Clasp your feet with your hands and bring them as close to your groin as is comfortable. Take a deep in-breath.*

*3. As you exhale, bend forward so that your head moves towards your feet.*

*4. Remain in this position for a few seconds, breathing gently, and focusing on the hara.*

*5. Slowly return to the sitting position on an in-breath.*

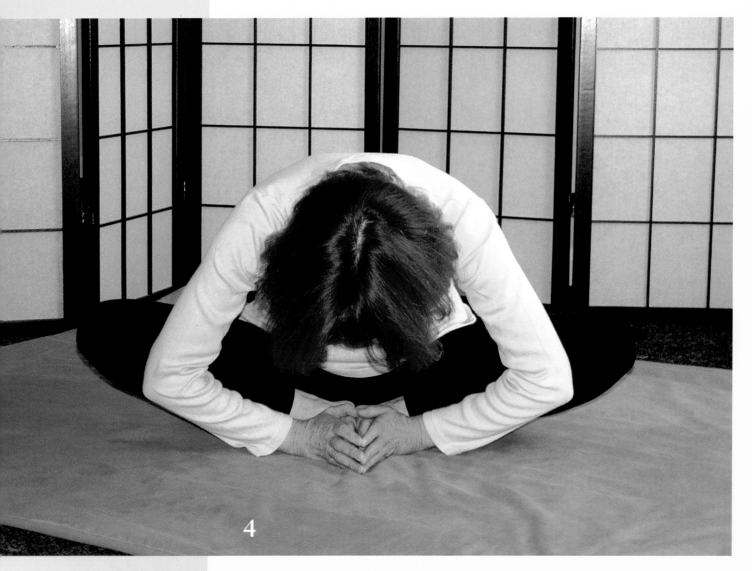

4

## EXERCISE 4 – HEART GOVERNOR/TRIPLE HEATER

These meridians relate to the FIRE element.

*1. Sit cross-legged on the floor, right leg on top of the left.*

*2. Cross your arms, left arm on top of the right, with your hands clasping your knees.*

*3. As you exhale, lean forward, pushing down on your knees.*

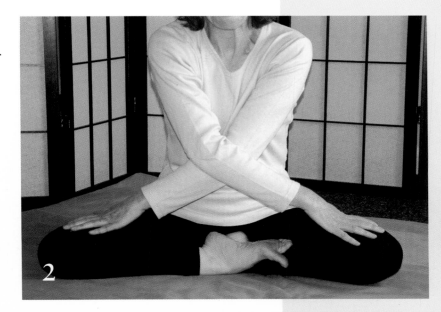

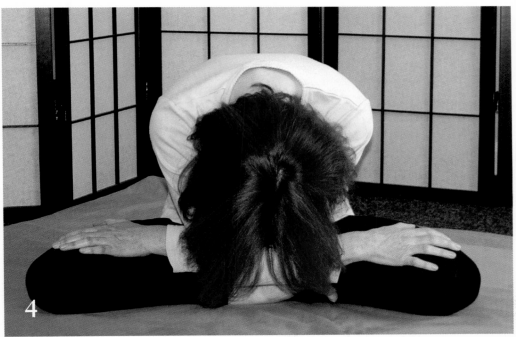

*4. Relax your neck and head and allow them to drop forward.*

*5. Remain in this position, breathing steadily.*

*6. Return to the starting position as you inhale.*

*7. Reverse the instructions for placing of the legs and arms and repeat the previous six steps.*

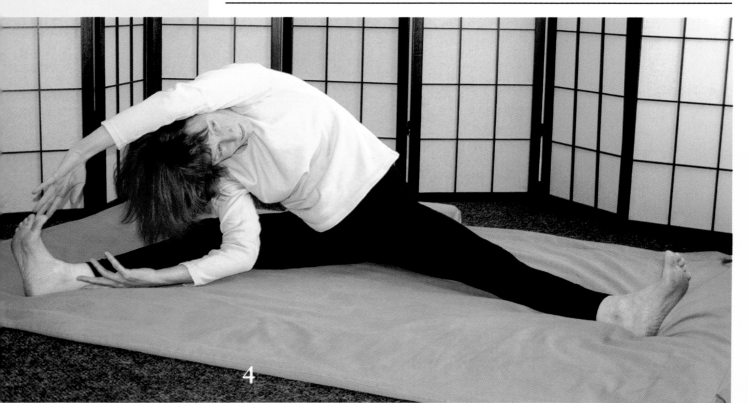

4

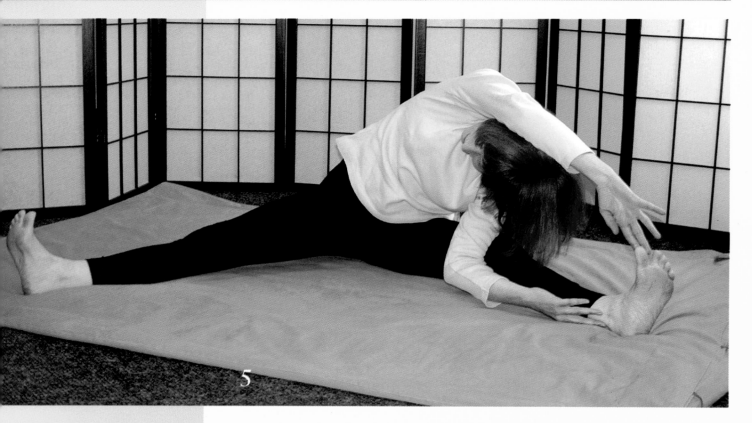

5

### EXERCISE 5 – BLADDER/KIDNEYS

These meridians relate to the WATER element.

*1. Sit on the floor, legs stretched out in front of you and close together.*

*2. Lean forward and reach out to clasp your feet. If you can't manage this, touch your ankles, shins – even your knees.*

*3. Allow your head to drop forward towards your knees.*

*4. Inhale as you slowly return to the sitting position.*

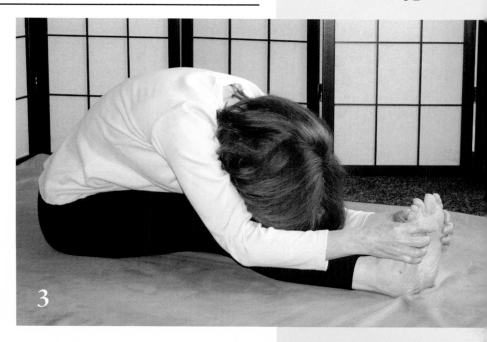

### EXERCISE 6 – LIVER/GALL BLADDER

These meridians relate to the WOOD element.

*1. Sit upright on the floor with your legs as wide apart as possible.*

*2. Stretch up your right arm, keeping the left arm at your side.*

*3. Now lean to the left and try to touch your left foot with your right hand.*

*4. Hold the stretch while breathing gently.*

*5. Return to the starting position, reverse the arms and repeat the exercise.*

*6. Next return to the first position, hands clasped in front of you.*

*7. Bend forward from the hips and relax into the stretch.*

*8. Return to the upright position.*

**Caution:** Unless you are very supple, you will probably find this exercise difficult at first. Persevere, but don't try to force anything.

**Rest and relax**
When you have completed this set of exercises, make a point of laying flat on the floor for several minutes. Close your eyes, breathe deeply and regularly, and relax.

*Above: exercise 5 – bladder/kidneys.*

*Far left: exercise 6 – liver/gall bladder.*

# YOU ARE WHAT YOU EAT

Over the past few decades, we have been swamped with information and advice about diet. There are all sorts of diets – most of them claiming to be the ultimate in healthy eating. But the decision about exactly what to eat is complicated by a number of other factors. We are warned about the effects of pollution, about the chemical sprays used on crops, the hormones fed to livestock, and about genetic modification, to name but a few of the hazards of putting food into our mouths. Then along came BSE and more recently Foot and Mouth Disease. In fact, many of us began to wonder if any food was safe to eat.

*Below: we are warned about the effects of pollution on the food we eat and it is worthwhile trying to combat any harm this may have on our bodies by eating as healthier a diet as possible.*

It is consoling, of course, to realise that the media as a whole tends to be alarmist. We don't have to accept as gospel every word we hear on television or read in the newspapers. At the same time, it's common sense to eat as healthily as circumstances permit. The only strict Shiatsu diet is the one advised for Macrobiotic Shiatsu and many people find this too restrictive. Even so, bearing in mind that this is an holistic discipline, it makes sense to consider what you eat and to make changes, if necessary.

## TAKE YOUR TIME

As with all other aspects of Shiatsu, you are advised to take a relaxed approach. Don't rush to make drastic changes in your diet. And whatever you eat, take your time about it. The all-too-common habit of eating "on the run" causes all sorts of digestive disturbances.

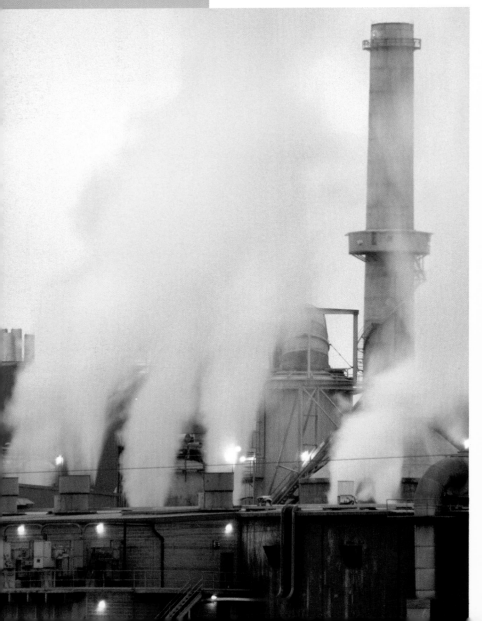

## THE IDEAL DIET

Some Shiatsu practitioners advise a typically Oriental diet, based on the Five Flavours – bitter, sweet, pungent, salty and sour. Others advise a balance of Yin and Yang foods. For the average Westerner, such considerations may seem somewhat complex and time-consuming. It is comparatively simple to work out a healthy diet from the following guidelines.

### EAT

**Grains** – whole wheat, brown rice, millet, oats etc.

**Fruit** – all fruits are valuable.

**Vegetables** – all vegetables, particularly the green variety.

**Pulses** – lentils, beans, chick peas etc.

**Nuts** – almonds, walnuts, cashews etc. (unless you suffer from nut allergy).

**Fish** – most types, but particularly oily fish such as mackerel, tuna and salmon.

**Meat** – restrict your intake. Poultry, such as chicken or turkey, is preferable to red meat.

**Dairy products** – skimmed or semi-skimmed milk, live yogurt, cheese (sparingly.)

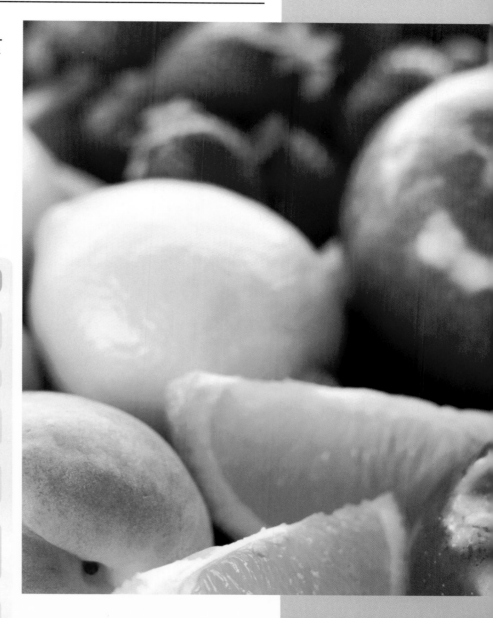

### DRINK

Herb teas, fruit teas, fruit and vegetable juices, and still bottled water. Try to drink at least four glasses of plain water every day, to begin with, then increase it gradually until you are drinking eight.

*Above: all fruits are valuable and should play a large part in the ideal diet*

## AVOID

Sugar (use honey as a substitute).
Salt (use herbs and spices instead).
"Fast food" – burgers, chips, etc.
Alcohol (though some dietitians
recommend a glass of good red
wine every day).
Red meat, sausages, etc.
Coffee, tea, cocoa, cola drinks.

*Below: avoid sugar and use honey as a substitute if absolutely necessary.*

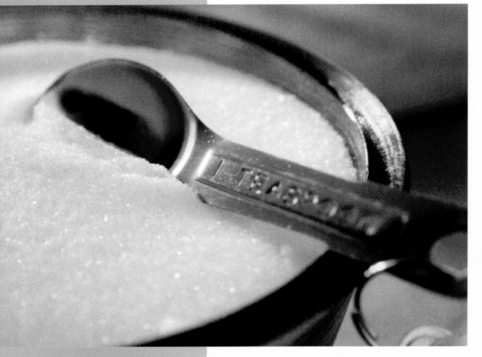

## WHAT CONSTITUTES A HEALTHY DIET?

A healthy diet is usually
considered to be made up as
follows.
- Whole grains     30/45%
- Vegetables       15/20%
- Fruit            15%
- Fats/sweets etc. 5% maximum

## THE HAY DIET

You may find that the Hay Diet is
convenient and easy to follow.
Briefly, it recommends that
carbohydrates – anything starchy
or sweet – should be eaten
separately from protein. It also
advises that carbohydrates and
protein should not be eaten within
four hours of each other. If you
have digestive problems, you may
find this diet helpful, since it
involves eating several small meals
a day rather than three large ones.

## WHAT ABOUT FOOD SUPPLEMENTS?

So far as Shiatsu is concerned,
there are no strict rules about this.
Some dietitians advocate a daily
dose of Vitamin C, others insist
that selenium is essential. The
most sensible course seems to be to
concentrate on eating a healthy
diet and practising Shiatsu. Then,
if you feel you have any problems
that could be solved by food
supplements consult a dietitian or
nutritionist. There is no point at
all in spending vast sums of money
on filling yourself up with pills
and potions. In fact, this could be
harmful since a number of
manufacturers recommend that
you take only a "course" of the
tablets – usually lasting about six
weeks.

Even if you have no intention of using Shiatsu to treat other people, do invest in at least one treatment by a qualified practitioner.

### FINDING A PRACTITIONER

Nowadays, professional organisations exist for most complementary therapies and Shiatsu is no exception. In the UK, the Shiatsu Society is the primary organisation, uniting students, teachers and practitioners (see Appendix.) You would be well advised to contact the Society to obtain details of a recognised Shiatsu practitioner in your area, rather than follow up advertisements in the local paper. Practitioners registered with the Shiatsu Society use the initials MRSS (Member of the Register of the Shiatsu Society) after their name.

### BEFORE THE APPOINTMENT

Having found a practitioner, ascertained his/her credentials and made an appointment, you will probably be given a few guidelines about your first experience of Shiatsu. You will be asked to wear just one layer of loose clothing in light, natural fabrics.

A cotton tee shirt and cargo trousers or jogging pants would be ideal.

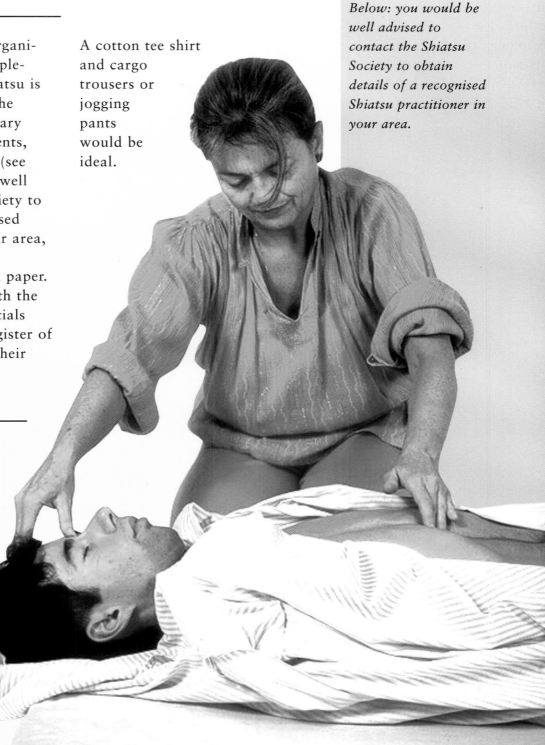

*Below: you would be well advised to contact the Shiatsu Society to obtain details of a recognised Shiatsu practitioner in your area.*

*Right: if at all possible, have a bath or a shower and put on clean clothing before keeping your appointment. This will relax you and help to calm any natural apprehension you may feel.*

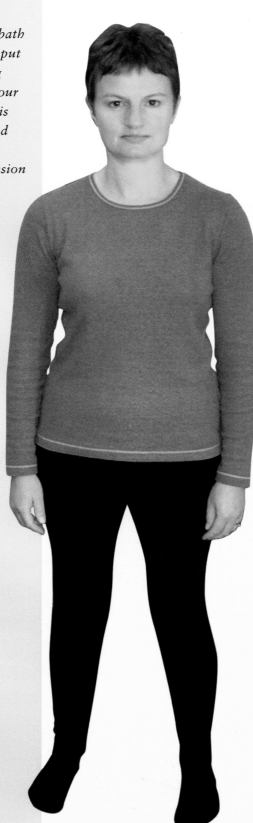

## SUITABLE CLOTHING

If at all possible, have a bath or a shower and put on clean clothing before keeping your appointment. This will relax you and help to calm any natural apprehension you may feel.

Try not to eat a large meal within two or three hours of the appointment. On the other hand, you will not be able to relax if you are hungry. A light snack about an hour before you leave the house is fine.

So now you're all ready to keep the appointment. What can you expect?

## PROFESSIONAL ASSESSMENT

Your first Shiatsu session will probably last an hour or more. The practitioner will need to make a detailed assessment of your current state of health before proceeding to offer treatment. This will enable them to diagnose the underlying cause of any problems you may have.

## DIAGNOSIS

In order to do this, the practitioner will almost certainly use one – or maybe all – of the four basic Shiatsu diagnostic categories. These are :

> **Observation**
>
> **Questioning**
>
> **Listening and smelling**
>
> **Touching**

## OBSERVATION

A trained Shiatsu practitioner will be able to learn a lot from simply looking at you. The lines on your face, the colours of your skin, your posture and general demeanour – even the clothes you are wearing – will all provide essential information about your health and state of mind. They will also have a look at your tongue, another important diagnostic area.

## QUESTIONING

You will be asked a variety of questions about your current and past state of health, any medication you are taking or have taken, and about your family's health. They will be interested in your likes and dislikes, your lifestyle, hopes, fears and worries.

Don't regard all these questions as a cross-examination. They are designed to give the practitioner a clear picture of your mental and physical health and your personality. In any case, all facts revealed during this type of consultation are strictly confidential and will not be revealed to any other person.

*Below: a trained Shiatsu practitioner will be able to learn a lot from simply looking at you.*

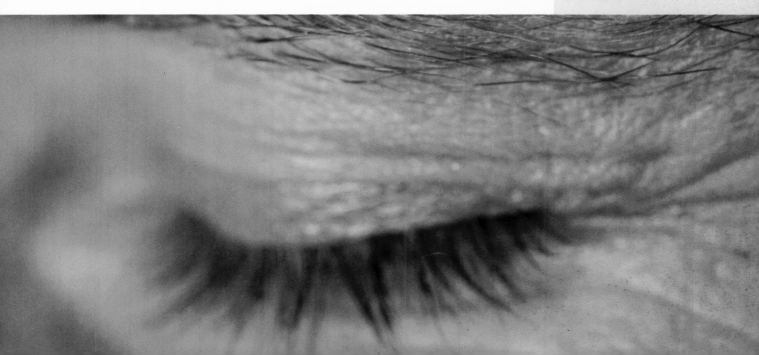

### LISTENING AND SMELLING

While you are answering questions and talking, the practitioner will also be noticing your tone of voice. According to the Five Elements theory there are five classifications.

> **Shouting**
>
> **Sing-song**
>
> **Monotonous**
>
> **Tearful**
>
> **Groaning**

*Below: a weak voice indicates a low Ki level and a strong one suggests the opposite – a strong Ki.*

As an example – if the practitioner detects a slightly tearful or "whiny" tone to your voice it could indicate that you are a metal-type person and that your lungs and large intestine meridians require attention. If you're inclined to shout, you may have a tendency to anger and this would indicate that liver and gall bladder meridians are involved.

As a rule of thumb, a weak voice indicates a low Ki level and a strong one suggests the opposite – a strong Ki. Please be sure to speak in your normal tone of voice. If you try to change it, you will merely mislead the practitioner.

The practitioner's sense of smell also comes into play here. It would be better not to wear perfume or after-shave when you go for your first treatment. Despite these aids, we each have our own distinctive odour and it is the practitioner's job to notice this. Don't feel embarrassed – after all, this is one of the ways in which our pet animals recognise us.

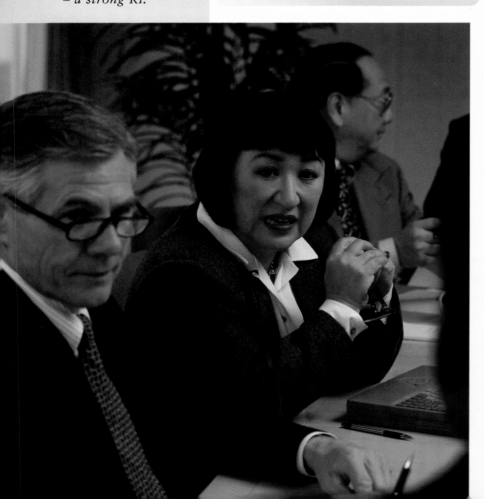

## TOUCHING

This is the most important of the Shiatsu diagnostic methods and the one on which the practitioner will probably spend most time.

There are certain areas of the body where an experienced practitioner can feel the quality of the Ki flowing through the meridians very clearly. They will, of course, ask your permission before touching you, but don't feel shy about this. It is by touching you that the practitioner will be most likely to be able to pinpoint the meridians that need most attention.

Now that the practitioner has made their assessment of your needs, what happens next?

### Basic Shiatsu Routine

In true Japanese style, some of the Shiatsu treatment will require you to lie on a mat or futon on the floor. At other times, you will sit up, probably supported by the practitioner.

Unlike some bodywork therapies, Shiatsu does not require the treatment to be carried out in any particular order. Most practitioners develop their own routine, but this may vary considerably in the light of what treatment the client requires. That being so, we list below the positions you will probably be required to adopt for treatment of meridians in various parts of the body.

> **Lying face down**
>
> **Lying on your back**
>
> **Lying on your side**
>
> **Sitting**

These four positions give the practitioner access to all the meridians requiring treatment. However, you should not expect your first treatment to involve all these positions. Having decided which meridians most need attention, the practitioner will position you accordingly.

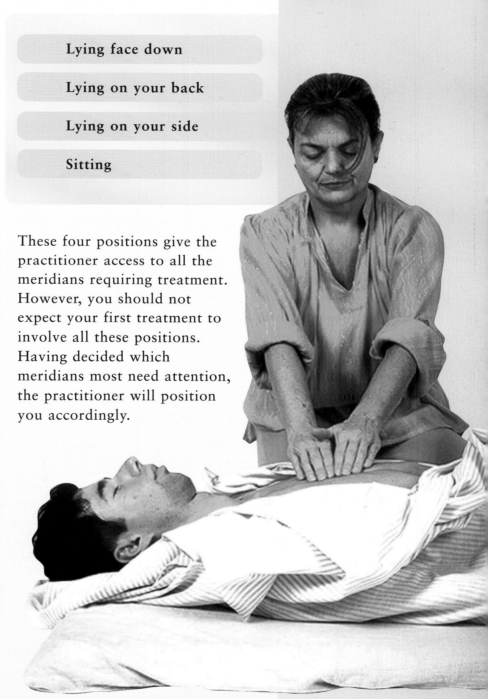

*Below: it is by touching you that the practitioner will be most likely to be able to pinpoint the meridians that need most attention.*

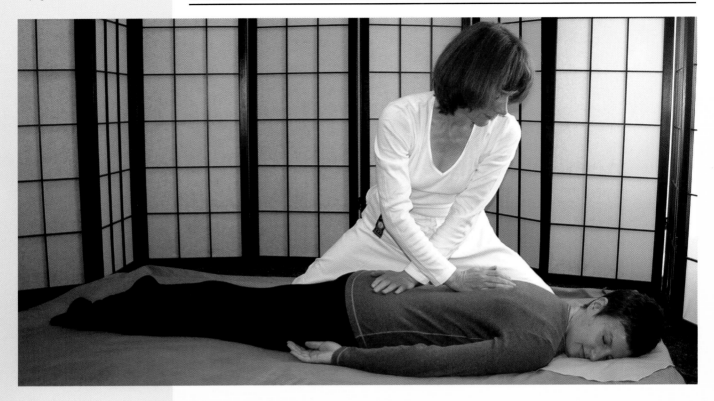

*Above: lying face down provides easy access to meridians at the back of the body and to the shoulders and back of the neck.*

## LYING FACE DOWN

Most people find it quite natural to lie in the prone position and, for this reason, the practitioner may well begin the treatment here.

This position provides easy access to meridians at the back of the body and to the shoulders and back of the neck, a common site for muscular tension. Channels accessible in this position include the bladder, small intestine and kidney meridians.

Your practitioner will probably begin the session by stretching your spine. They will use both hands for this, one at the top of the spine and one in the lumbar region.

The next step will involve work on the bladder meridian, which has two pathways, one on either side of the spine. This may be followed by the application of various types of pressure as they work down your back and on your shoulders.

Work on your legs will include treatment on the thighs, the backs of the knees and the calves. The practitioner may also use a leg-bending routine.

## LYING ON YOUR BACK

When you are asked to lie on your back, don't be surprised if you suddenly feel vulnerable and slightly uneasy. This position exposes the chest and the abdomen, the two main physical centres of the emotions. You will probably notice that the practitioner takes particular care to ensure that you are comfortable and to reassure you by adopting a gentle approach.

They may also regulate their breathing pattern to the same rhythm as your own and is unlikely to start any treatment until they are quite sure that you are relaxed and ready to be touched.

Before working on your arms and shoulders, they may gently shake the arm on which they are working until it feels loose and soft. Don't worry if, at first, you feel slightly apprehensive. This is natural and the tension will gradually ease as the session continues.

In this supine position, too, work will be done on your hips and legs. Sometimes, the practitioner may use their elbow on the outer thighs. If you find this uncomfortable in any way, say so immediately and they will use palm pressure. The hips and legs routine also involves lifting your knees and gently rotating the hip joints.

Most clients find the Shiatsu routine for face, head and neck extremely pleasant and relaxing. It begins when the practitioner cradles your head in their hands and very gently lifts and pulls your neck joints. Next they will roll your head from side to side and then conclude the treatment with gentle fingertip pressure on the contours of your face.

*Below: lying on your back exposes the chest and the abdomen, the two main physical centres of the emotions.*

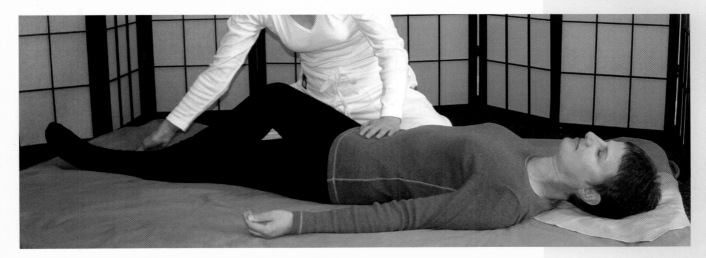

## LYING ON YOUR SIDE

It is important that you should feel comfortable in this position, so make sure of this before the practitioner begins treatment.

They will probably open this part of the session by rotating your arm and shoulder joint. This will be followed by stretching, but they will be watching closely to ensure that you are not experiencing any discomfort.

*Below: it is important that you should feel comfortable when lying on your side.*

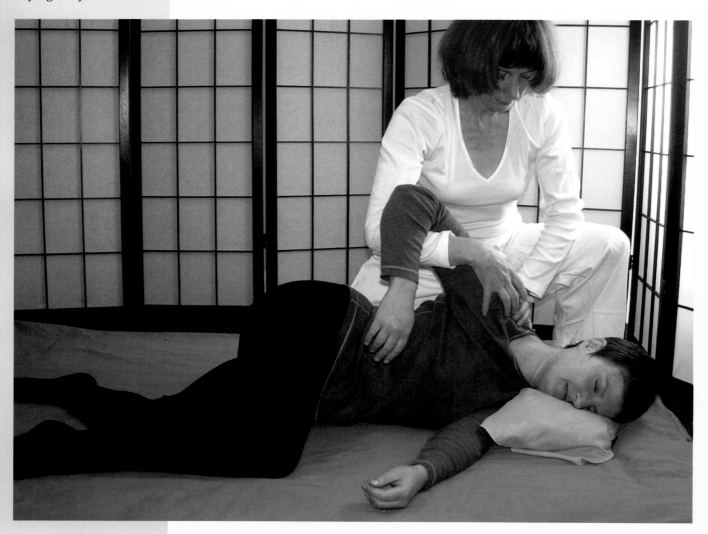

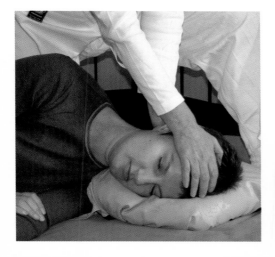

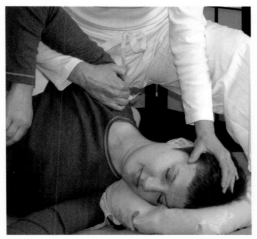

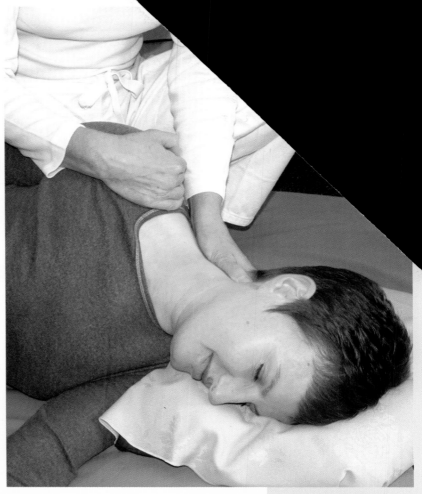

## WORK ON THE SIDE OF THE HEAD

When they begin to work on the side of your head, the practitioner will use gentle palm pressure and will also work along the base of your skull with their thumbs. The pressure used may vary, but do protest at once if you find it uncomfortable.

Work on the head is particularly important as it helps to balance the Yin and Yang energies.

Other routines employed while the client is in this position include treatment of the outer arm and hands, side stretches and attention to the inner and outer leg.

*Above: work on the head is particularly important as it helps to balance the Yin and Yang energies.*

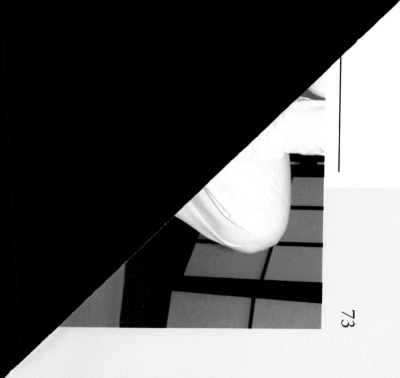

ive a

a

his.

ding
ts of
ber
ever
a

73

The obvious sitting position, of course, is on an ordinary kitchen or dining chair. Alternatively, you may sit astride the chair, facing the back of it. Some people like to sit on a stool, enabling the practitioner to approach them from all angles.

You may prefer to sit cross-legged on the floor or to kneel, but in both of these positions you will probably need to get up and stretch from time to time. Your practitioner will be happy to accommodate any position you prefer.

Obviously, sitting positions permit easy access to the back and shoulders. The practitioner may use their palms, their forearms or their elbows during this part of the treatment. As always – remember to complain immediately you feel any pain or discomfort.

Neck and back stretches are also involved here. In fact, most of the back treatments carried out when the client is lying face down can also be given in the sitting position.

**At the end of the treatment**
When the treatment is completed, the practitioner may sit at your head, resting their hands on your forehead. After a few moments, they will gently remove their hands, cover you with a light blanket and ask you to relax for a while.

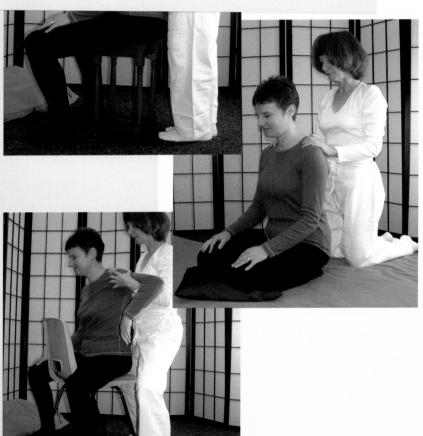

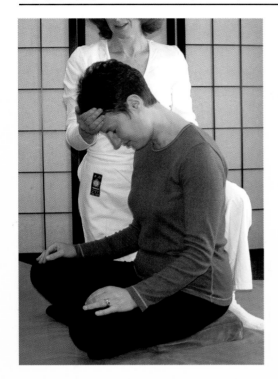

## RESTING AFTER TREATMENT

Don't rush this procedure. You may well be feeling "spaced out" and should not move until you feel completely ready to do so.

Some practitioners advise clients not to drive immediately after treatment. This is something to bear in mind if you feel even slightly light-headed or shaky. Sit comfortably, relax and take some deep breaths.

There is no need to hurry. The practitioner will certainly not have another client champing at the bit in their waiting room. Take your time and make the most of your first experience of Shiatsu.

## AFTER EFFECTS

In the days following your first treatment, you may experience a few mild reactions. This is because Shiatsu clears toxins from the body into the blood stream, and this may aggravate your symptoms for a day or two. Don't worry about this. Drink lots of water, rest as much as possible and you will soon feel the full benefit of the treatment.

## HOW MANY SESSIONS?

A lot of people experience such a tremendous sense of well-being from their first Shiatsu treatment that they continue to make appointments, even if this is not necessary. That's fine and will certainly be beneficial, though it can prove expensive. The usual recommendation for a course of treatment is between four and eight sessions at weekly intervals, but much depends on the client's progress.

*Left: when the treatment is completed, the practitioner may sit at your head, resting their hands on your forehead.*

*Below: after a few moments, they will gently remove their hands, cover you with a light blanket and ask you to relax for a while.*

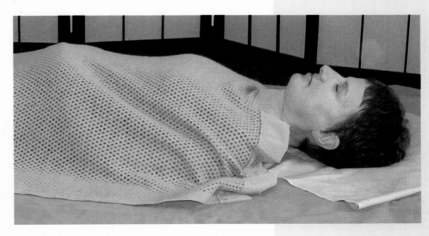

# SELF-TREATMENT

There will be times when – however much you would like to have a professional Shiatsu treatment – this is out of the question. However, it is always possible to adapt Shiatsu techniques for self-treatment. One advantage of such self-treatment is that it gives you experience in locating pressure points. In treating yourself, too, you will learn at first hand just how much pressure is required.

Obviously, you will not be able to reach all the pressure points when treating yourself, but it is easy to adapt the techniques for the front of the body, the arms and legs.

*Right: it is easy to adapt the techniques for the front of the body, the arms and legs.*

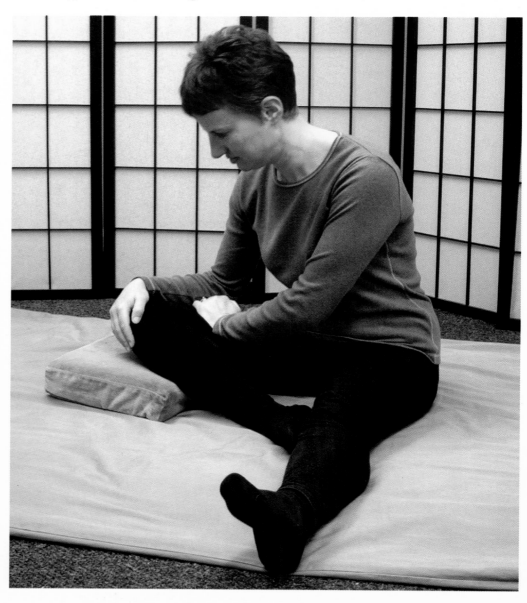

# SELF-TREATMENT TECHNIQUES

### HEADACHES

Apply gentle pressure in the hollow at the inside of the upper eye socket.

### ONE-SIDED HEADACHES, TENSION AND NECK PAIN

Find the hollow at the back of the neck, just under the skull and between the two large neck muscles. Apply gentle thumb pressure.

### INTESTINAL PROBLEMS

Apply pressure on top of the forearm muscles, about three finger widths down from the elbow crease in the inside of the arm. This is also helpful to ease pain in the shoulders.

### CONSTIPATION, DIARRHOEA, TOOTHACHE AND HEADACHES

Apply pressure close to the bones on the web between the thumb and index finger.

### TRAVEL SICKNESS

Apply pressure on the inner arm, two thumb widths above the wrist crease and between the tendons. This pressure point will also control vomiting.

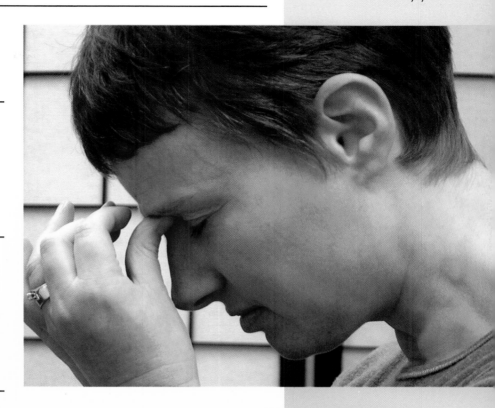

### HYSTERIA

Apply pressure on the inside corner of the cuticle of one of your finger nails.

### EXHAUSTION AND LACK OF VITALITY

Flex your index finger and bend it forward to touch a point in the palm of your hand. Apply pressure to this point for 15 seconds.

### SINUS TROUBLE AND NASAL CONGESTION

Press inwards and upwards on the spaces under your cheekbones, directly beneath the pupils of the eyes when staring straight ahead.

*Above: apply gentle pressure in the hollow at the inside of the upper eye socket for relief of headaches.*

## FLATULENCE, DISTENSION, DIGESTIVE DISCOMFORT

Spread the right hand, exposing the web between the thumb and the index finger. Place the left thumb on the back of the web and the index finger on the other side. Apply gentle massage for a few seconds, then repeat the process on the left hand.

**NB:** *This remedy should not be used if you are pregnant.*

## LOW BACK PAIN

With the index finger, apply firm pressure to the indentation above the upper lip and beneath the nostrils.

These are just a few of the Shiatsu techniques that can be employed as first aid remedies for yourself and, of course, for other people. As you become more experienced in using Shiatsu techniques, you will be able to adapt several more for self-treatment.

Remember, too, that the Do-In exercises and the Makko-ho stretches are effective in dispersing various minor aches and pains. They are also particularly valuable for the relief of stress.

**NB:** *The Shiatsu remedies listed here are strictly First Aid treatments. Should the symptoms worsen or persist for several days, you should make an appointment to see your doctor.*

*Below: for lower back pain apply firm pressure to the indentation above the upper lip and beneath the nostrils using the index finger.*

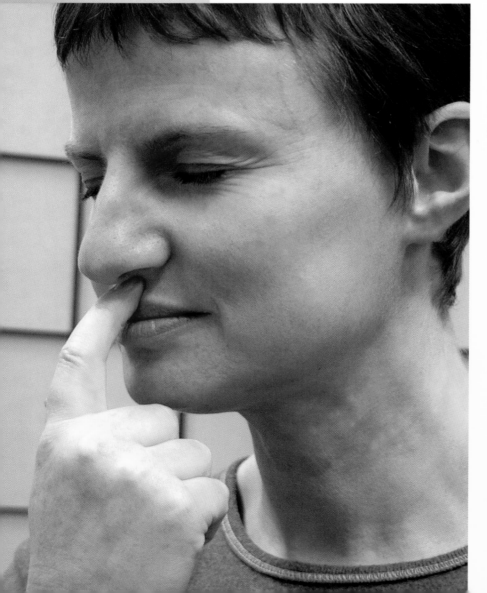

Shiatsu is not a cure-all. There are undoubtedly many conditions on which it will have little, if any, effect. Even so, there are a number of everyday ailments that can be alleviated by Shiatsu treatment. Because Shiatsu uses the holistic approach, you may find that your emotional and spiritual condition improves after treatment, even if the physical symptoms remain.

## CAUTION NEEDED

It is a mistake to rush into giving (or receiving) Shiatsu treatment without first considering the condition involved. There are times when Shiatsu is definitely inappropriate and could even be harmful.

For example, during the **first three months** of pregnancy the use of certain pressure points can increase the risk of a miscarriage. Later in pregnancy, Shiatsu treatment can be relaxing and helpful, but it should always be administered by a qualified practitioner.

**Contagious or infectious diseases** may or may not respond to Shiatsu treatment, but in any case it is not a good idea to be in physical contact with anyone suffering from such illnesses. It is wise to postpone treatment until all risk of infection has passed.

**Skin problems** can present the same risk of transferring infection. Additionally, even the lightest touch on the affected area may be too painful. This applies, too, to

most **burns, bruises and lesions**. For obvious reasons, you should not apply pressure of any kind to **fractures, broken bones or damaged muscles**. Varicose veins are another no-go area, where pressure would be extremely painful and could cause damage.

However, even if it is not possible to give treatment to the affected area, Shiatsu at certain pressure points elsewhere on the body can provide a calming and soothing effect that will alleviate the physical discomfort.

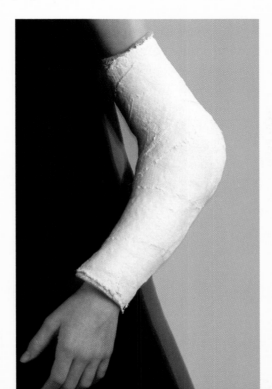

*Left: you should not apply pressure of any kind to fractures, broken bones or damaged muscles.*

### WHAT SHIATSU CAN HELP

Many of the everyday ailments that beset us nowadays are caused by stress, tension and overwork. In these circumstances, Shiatsu is the ideal treatment. It is also effective as a self-help tool in dealing with a number of minor physical conditions.

The aim of Shiatsu is to restore balance and strength to your body. When you feel "under the weather" for any reason, Shiatsu can calm your agitation, relax tension and stimulate the flow of Ki in your body to renew your vitality.

### SHIATSU CAN

- *balance body, mind and spirit;.*
- *relieve stress and tension;*
- *calm over-emotional reactions;*
- *relieve indigestion;*
- *help menstrual difficulties;*
- *increase energy levels;*
- *produce deep relaxation;*
- *alleviate minor aches and pains;*
- *treat a variety of everyday ailments;*
- *relieve migraine and other headaches.*

### BREATHING

All the above conditions and many others can be eased by one of Shiatsu's most effective tools – the breath. Deep breathing is energising. Shallow breathing produces a nervous reaction and lacks vitality.

Breathing correctly is particularly useful as part of dealing with any form of distress, emotional or physical. Deep inhalation stimulates the flow of Ki throughout your body. Exhalation is powerfully relaxing.

It is especially beneficial if you and the person giving the Shiatsu treatment can breathe in unison. This is known as co-ordinated breathing.

### WHO BENEFITS FROM SHIATSU?

Everybody can benefit from Shiatsu treatment. Surprisingly, it also works very well for the "touch me not" people who dislike personal contact. If they can agree to just one Shiatsu session, they often find that they are released from the phobia.

As was said earlier, Shiatsu is not a cure-all or a universal panacea, but it will have a beneficial effect on practically every condition known to man (or woman, for that matter.)

## SHIATSU FOR CHILDREN

Quite apart from its undoubted healing functions, Shiatsu is of tremendous benefit to children in several ways. First, if the treatment is administered by the parent, it enhances and strengthens the parent/child bond. Second, children invariably enjoy Shiatsu treatment. In this way it can be a means of treating some slight ailment without the child even realising it. And third, it enables the parent to notice and, if necessary, question the child about any injuries or slight abnormalities.

Children who are hyperactive or difficult respond particularly well to Shiatsu treatment, if they can be persuaded to submit to it for the first time. Thereafter, there is seldom any problem. They enjoy being the centre of attention and find the treatment very relaxing.

## HOW MUCH PRESSURE?

When treating babies under the age of two, no pressure should be used. Instead, use a gentle stroking action. This will be equally effective and will probably soothe the child to sleep. Between the ages of two and five, some very slight pressure may be permissible – much depending on the child's reaction – but stroking and

rubbing are probably best. After the age of five, the usual Shiatsu techniques can be used, provided you remember that you **are** treating a child, not an adult. You will, of course, always bear in mind any handicaps or illnesses from which the child may suffer. For example, children with cerebral palsy respond well to Shiatsu. Administering the treatment will require great patience from the practitioner, but Shiatsu is a valuable means of reducing muscular spasms in these children.

Watsu Shiatsu (treatment in a pool of warm water) has proved to be especially effective for disabled children.

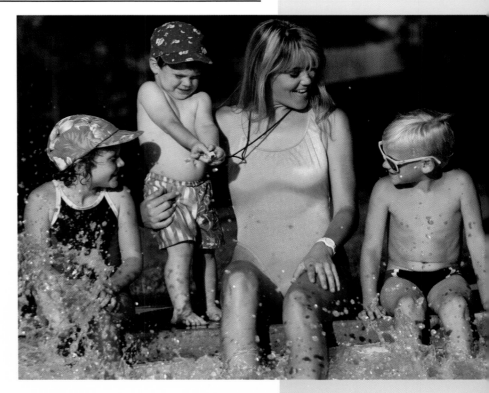

*Above: Shiatsu is of tremendous benefit to children.*

### SHIATSU FOR THE ELDERLY

*Below: Shiatsu can be particularly helpful in many of the conditions associated with increasing age.*

*Far right: most people tend to wait until a health problem develops before they seek medical help.*

Shiatsu can be particularly helpful in many of the conditions associated with increasing age. Here, as with children, the practitioner needs to be wary of exerting too much pressure. Sometimes, no pressure at all is needed. Older people will respond as happily as children to gentle, stroking movements.

What is termed the "touchy-feely" approach is apt to be scornfully dismissed, but the fact remains that sensory stimulation is essential to our good health.

This sort of human contact is vitally important to older people, and gentle Shiatsu treatment is an ideal way of providing it. When you're feeling depressed or "under the weather", nothing is more encouraging than a warm-hearted hug from a friend. This can be a pleasant way to end a Shiatsu treatment for an older person.

Because Shiatsu treatment enhances the flow of Ki throughout the body, older people usually find it a physically stimulating experience that may help to alleviate any pain they are suffering. Similarly, they feel more alert and optimistic as a result of the emotional and mental effects of the treatment. Finally – and possibly most important – regular Shiatsu treatment is an effective palliative for insomnia.

### WHY SHIATSU?

According to a recent report from the Shiatsu Society and the Research Council for Complementary Medicine, people seek Shiatsu treatment mainly for neck, shoulder and back pain or for arthritis. The second most common reasons were stress, anxiety and depression.

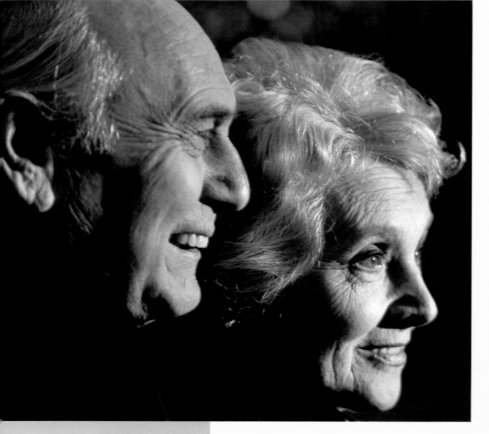

## PREVENTION IS BETTER THAN CURE

Although Shiatsu is principally regarded as a healing method, it can also be used as a preventative therapy. In the rush and bustle of everyday life, most people tend to wait until a health problem develops before they seek medical help.

*"It will go away," they say, hopefully.*

Obviously, this is a mistake. The ailment seldom goes away. It is much more likely to increase in severity.

The ideal, of course, would be to receive regular weekly Shiatsu treatment, but few can afford the time or the money involved. However, if you learn the basics of the therapy you will be able to use it on yourself and also to help friends and family. Even five minutes of Shiatsu a day can be an effective means of staying healthy.

By all means, have a professional Shiatsu treatment as often as you can, but supplement it with your own efforts. Your reward will be a sense of fulfilment and well-being that will go a long way towards alleviating the minor aches and pains and worries of life.

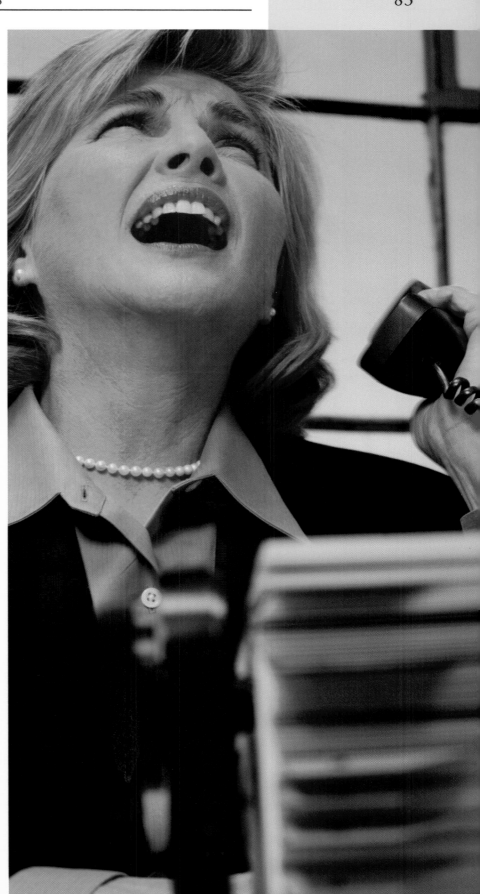

# BECOMING A PRACTITIONER

*Below: local authorities have started to offer classes in Shiatsu for beginners. Usually, the tutor is a qualified Shiatsu therapist.*

Becoming a professional Shiatsu practitioner/teacher is not a decision to be taken lightly. Having read so far in this book, you will be under no illusions about the degree of commitment required to attain professional status. So don't rush into this decision.

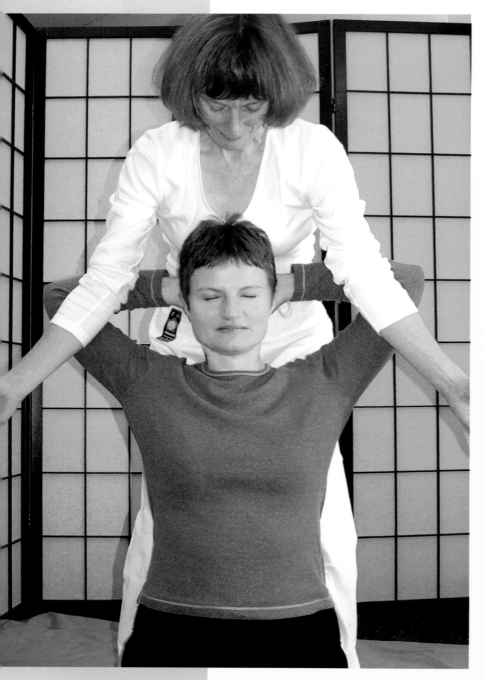

## ATTEND CLASSES

Over the past few years, a number of local authorities have started to offer classes in Shiatsu for beginners. Usually, the tutor is a qualified Shiatsu therapist and the classes are held in the evenings at a reasonable cost.

These classes will not qualify you to become a professional practitioner, but they will provide you with a clear insight into Shiatsu therapy. The tutor, too, will be able to give you some idea of how much commitment, time and money is required if you wish to take professional training.

## SHIATSU SCHOOLS

An increasing number of Shiatsu schools offer various types of training and you may find details of these in health magazines or "New Age" publications. Most of these courses are held at weekends, though one or two of the larger colleges offer full-time training. These courses are likely to be expensive and you would be wise to attend evening classes first to ascertain that you really do want to become a professional practitioner.

### FINDING A LOCAL TEACHER

You may find that there is a Shiatsu practitioner in your locality who will be prepared to accept you as a pupil. Be cautious here. No matter how well-qualified this person may be, he/she may not be a good teacher. In these circumstances, your best plan is to contact the Shiatsu Society to find out if this particular practitioner is also registered with them as a teacher.

### THE SHIATSU SOCIETY

This is the foremost Shiatsu organisation in the UK and, as such, can offer a great deal of help and advice. It demands high standards from the practitioners and teachers on its professional register. Before a practitioner can apply to join the teachers' register, they must have spent a minimum of two years in professional practice. And, having achieved teacher status, they must have been registered with the Society for five years before they can become principal of a school.

The address and telephone number of the Shiatsu Society appear in the Appendix. You will find the staff extremely helpful – and, incidentally, the Society also publishes a useful newsletter for members.

### QUALITIES REQUIRED

If you aspire to become a Shiatsu practitioner, you need to be sure that you possess the essential qualities involved – self-discipline, a caring attitude, patience and sensitivity.

You will also need to be truly enthusiastic about Shiatsu therapy and prepared to expend a great deal of time and concentration on learning about it. Most classes major on hands-on practice and this, of course, is important. But be prepared, too, for lessons in Traditional Chinese Medicine, physiology, anatomy and similar subjects.

*Above: be prepared for lessons in Traditional Chinese Medicine.*

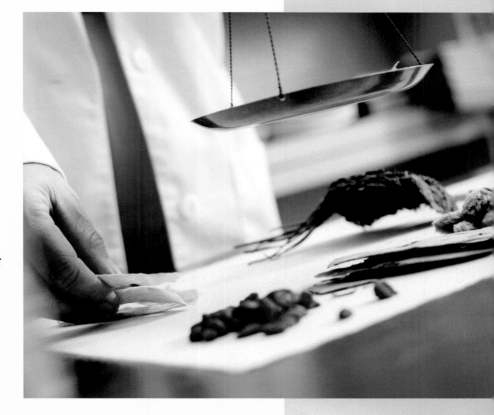

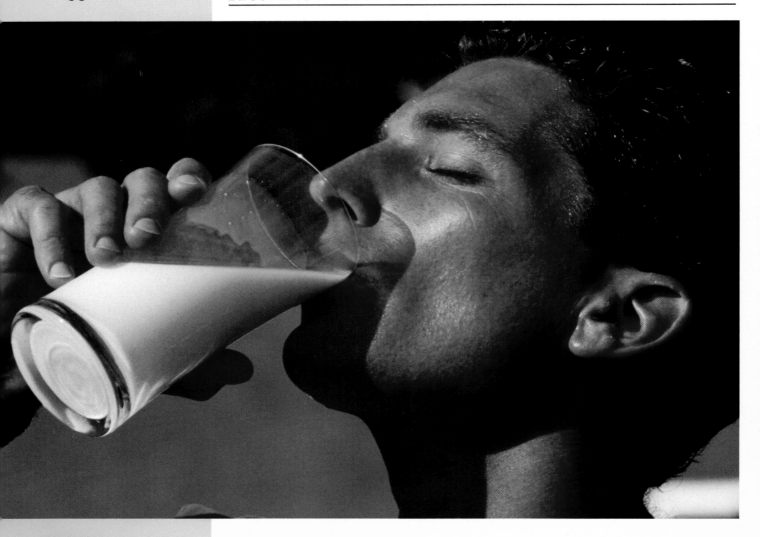

*Above: Shiatsu training will undoubtedly change your whole life and you will become more aware of the need for a healthy mind in a healthy body.*

## A DIFFERENT WAY OF LIFE

In short, undertaking Shiatsu training will undoubtedly change your whole life. Quite apart from the commitment to learning required, you will soon discover that you have developed a different outlook. Your emotional attitudes change as you learn to "tune in" to other people. You become more aware of the need for "a healthy mind in a healthy body". You adopt a more positive attitude. And perhaps, most important of all, you view other people in a completely different – and more compassionate – manner.

Becoming a Shiatsu practitioner will undoubtedly open for you a doorway to a completely new life. Be sure that this is what you want.

Shiatsu is an holistic therapy. This means that it affects every aspect of your life. If it is your intention to practise Shiatsu, now is the time to take stock of your lifestyle and to decide what changes – if any – need to be made.

We have already discussed the importance of healthy eating. Now we turn to two other essentials for good health – exercise and sleep.

## EXERCISE

You are already aware of the value of Do-In and Makko-ho exercises, but please try to incorporate other forms of physical activity into your way of life, too. If you already enjoy visiting a gym several times a week, that's fine. If the gym scene is not for you, consider taking a brisk 30-minute walk every day. Cycling, swimming, golf, badminton, squash – even line dancing – are other options. These and other forms of aerobic exercise will be of immense benefit to your cardio-vascular system.

If you don't have the time for an exercise session every day, try to increase the effort and vigour you use as you go about your daily life. Walk (briskly) instead of driving; run up the stairs at work, rather than using the lift; put extra effort into pushing the vacuum cleaner over the floor or mowing the lawn. In short – try to move twice as quickly as usual and put 100% more effort into everything you do.

The plus factor in all this is that you'll very quickly begin to enjoy a heightened sense of vitality and well-being. Your breathing and your appetite will improve and you'll be healthily tired so that you sleep well at night.

## SLEEP

If you happen to be an insomniac, you'll probably grin wryly at the previous statement. Nonetheless, it's true. Try an experiment for a month. Gradually increase your physical activity, get into the fresh air as much as you can and see how your sleep pattern has changed at the end of that time.

*Below: try to incorporate other forms of physical activity into your way of life, too.*

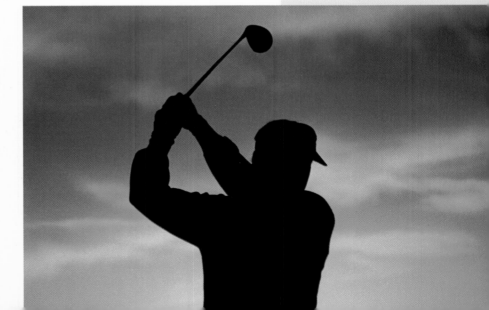

## INSOMNIA

*Below: to help combat insomnia have a warm drink and immerse yourself in an interesting book.*

What if you're one of those unfortunate people who have real sleeping problems? The least helpful thing you can do is worry about it. Don't lay in bed, tossing and turning and fretting about when you'll get to sleep.

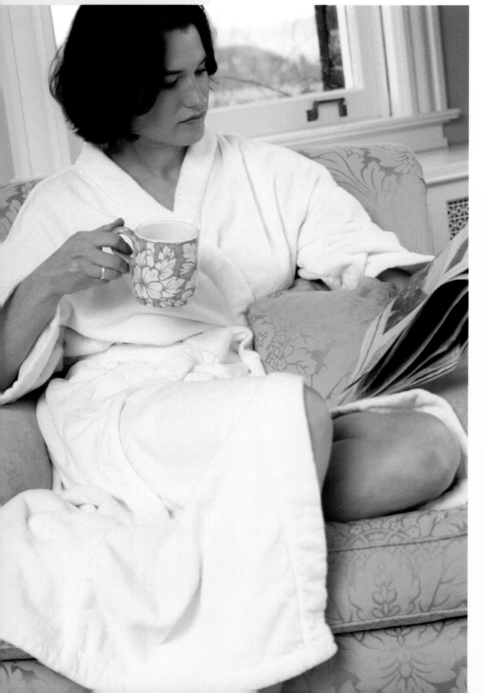

The answer is – you won't! It's far better to get up, have a warm drink and immerse yourself in an interesting book or watch late-night television.

When you begin to feel drowsy – and you will – go back to bed and relax as completely as possible. To do this, there's no need to follow the lengthy "talking to your big toe" routine. Simply tense every muscle in your body, hold the tension for a few seconds and then f-l-o-p!

Repeat this procedure a few times, then make yourself comfortable, close your eyes and begin to breathe rhythmically and quietly. You will drift softly into a deep sleep.

One more point. Don't expect immediate results. You need to persevere with this routine. There's no need to feel disheartened if you don't get instant results or if you have the occasional relapse. Take heart from the sure and certain knowledge that your new regime of fresh air/healthy eating/exercise – and, of course, Shiatsu – will pay off in the form of restful slumber.

## WHAT'S IT ALL ABOUT?

You're probably thinking that there's more to a full and happy life than the topics we have discussed here. This, of course, is true. Exactly **what** you need in order to have a satisfying life is very much a matter of individual choice.

A happy family life, a rewarding job, good friends – all these are important but, for each one of us, there is a certain emotional/spiritual requirement that will ensure a truly balanced and fulfilling life.

Do you have any idea of what your own personal need is? Probably not – but one of the truly magical properties of Shiatsu is that you will begin to find out. Yet again – don't rush at it. Don't devour every self-help book you can find or spend hours in search of the one balancing factor needed to make your life complete. Whatever that quality is, it will eventually become apparent to you.

## BAD HABITS

Most of us have developed a few habits that are not exactly conducive to good physical, mental and emotional health. Resolve to dispense with any that could deplete your energy, and to cultivate those that increase the flow of Ki throughout your body.

Sit down with a pen and paper and make a list of the habits you would like to eradicate from your life. Read through the list, crossing off each habit as you come to it. Then tear the paper in little pieces and tip them into the kitchen bin, saying a firm "Get lost!" as you close the lid.

This may sound crazy, but it works. You won't lose all your bad habits at once, but this is a good way to begin the process. It is also an excellent start to living your life the Shiatsu way.

Traditional Chinese Medicine claims that the main requirement for good health is balance – in body, mind and spirit and between all three. This same holistic approach underlies many other complementary therapies – yoga, reflexology, Tai Chi, – and, of course, Shiatsu.

*Far right: your mind is alert and active throughout every waking hour. Reading is important go to the library and borrow a book on a subject you've never even heard of. All this expands your brain's capacity to learn.*

## SHIATSU AND THE HOLISTIC APPROACH

At first, you may think that Shiatsu is concerned solely with the physical body. This is not so. Correctly applied, the bodily aspects of the therapy cannot fail to affect the recipient's mind and spirit, too.

Working with the meridians and pressure points undoubtedly eases pain and stiffness and, in so doing, promotes physical relaxation. This, in turn, eases mental worry and stress. And when both body and mind are at peace, we have time and space for spiritual matters.

We have already suggested various dietary changes that will enhance your physical health. Take time, too, to consider the health of your mental and spiritual systems. Your mind and spirit, as well as your body, need to be fed, if the ultimate experience of perfect balance is to be achieved.

## FEEDING THE MIND

Enhancing your mental health does not involve long periods of study. Realise, first of all, that your mind is alert and active throughout every waking hour. Make the most of this by taking notice of everything around you.

When did you last stop to watch an ant go zealously about its business?

Do you watch documentary programmes on television? They provide much food for thought. Quiz programmes and game shows can be equally stimulating on a different level.

Reading is important, too. If you've always read one national newspaper, try another. Go to the library and borrow a book on a subject you've never even heard of. All this expands your brain's capacity to learn.

It doesn't much matter **what** you watch or do or read. What is important is to be aware of what you are learning from these activities. Too often, we tend to sit in front of the television set in a sort of daze – vaguely aware of moving shadows on the screen, but not really absorbing anything very much.

The stimulation resulting from Shiatsu treatment will enhance your ability to focus on everything you see, hear and do.

You will grow in appreciation of the wonders all around you as you go about your daily life. As time goes by, you will realise that your mind is more active – and in better health – than ever before.

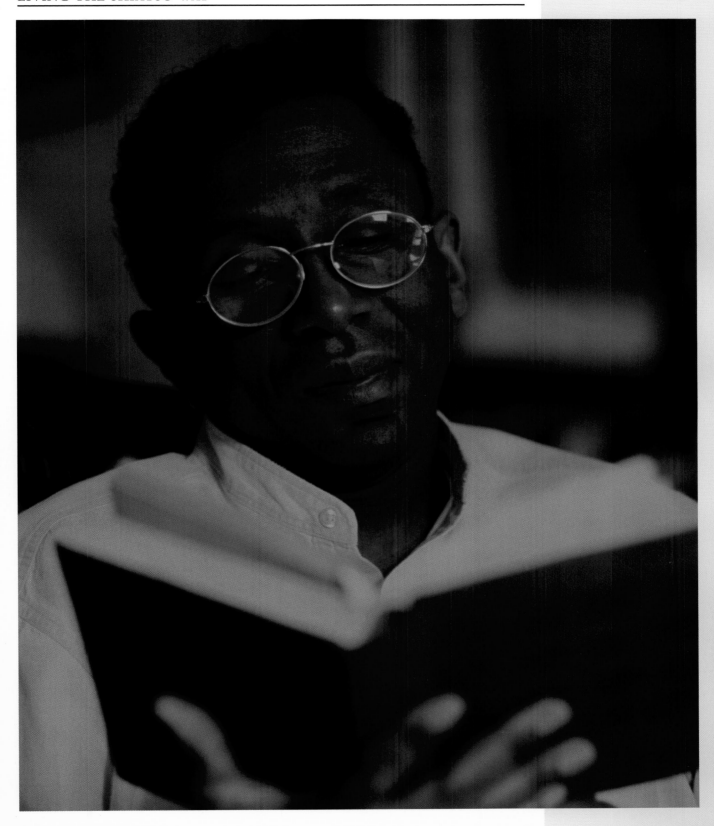

*Below: "spiritual" can be used to refer to religion and worship.*

## THE SPIRITUAL DIMENSION

In the context of Shiatsu, it doesn't matter whether you subscribe to a particular religion or none. The holistic approach requires only that body, mind and spirit are balanced – in other words, that each can live happily with the others. A healthy body with a calm and alert mind will eventually lead you to recognition of your spiritual self.

The term "spiritual" means different things to different people. It can be used to refer to religion and worship, to the soul, to music, art, beauty, nature; all these definitions – and many others – are correct. Your own particular spiritual dimension is exactly what you choose it to be.

As you learn more about Shiatsu and experience its many benefits, you may well discover your "inner self" – the essential you. This is not usually a sudden miraculous experience. The certainty that there is a spiritual aspect to you and to your life comes quietly and gradually. When it does arrive, you will know that you have achieved that much-desired harmony of body, mind and spirit – the greatest gift Shiatsu has to offer.

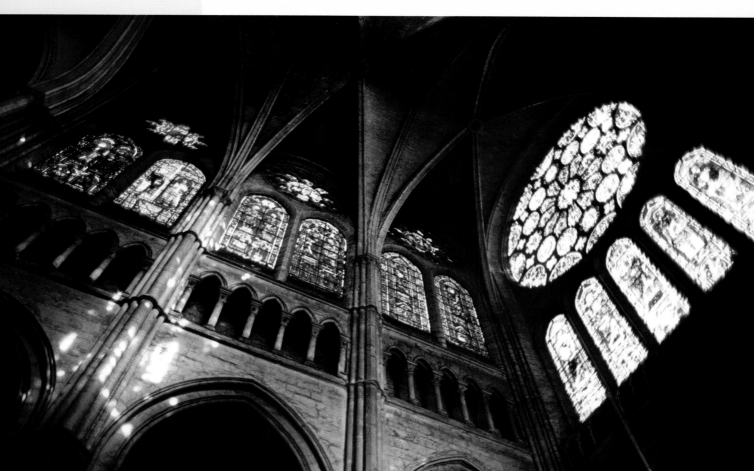

# APPENDIX

## USEFUL ADDRESSES

The Shiatsu Society
Eastland Court
St Peters Road
Rugby CV21 3QP

Telephone: 01758 555051
Fax: 01758 555052
Website: www.shiatsu.org

The Shiatsu College
20a Lower Goat Lane
Norwich NR2 1EL

Telephone: 01603 632555
Fax: 01603 663391

The European Shiatsu School
Central Administration
High Banks
Lockeridge
Marlborough
Wilts SN8 4EQ

Telephone: 01672 513444

Shiatsu International
31 Fletton Avenue
Peterborough PE2 8AX

Freephone: 0800 092 7091

## FURTHER READING

SHIATSU: The Complete Guide
Chris Jarmey and Gabriel Mojay
(Thorsons)

THE SHIATSU MANUAL
Gerry Thompson (Headline)

THE PRINCIPLES OF SHIATSU
Chris Jarmey (Thorsons)

HEALTH ESSENTIALS: SHIATSU
Elaine Liechti (Element Books)

SECRETS OF SHIATSU
Cathy Meeus (Dorling Kindersley)

THE BOOK OF SHIATSU
Paul Lundberg (Gaia Books)

A BEGINNER'S GUIDE TO
SHIATSU
Jane Downer (Hodder and
Stoughton)

THE THEORY AND PRACTICE
OF SHIATSU
Carola Beresford-Cook (Churchill
Livingstone)

# INDEX

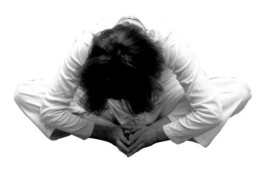